BETTER UNDERSTANDING OF THE CAMPYLOBACTER CONUNDRUM

BETTER UNDERSTANDING OF THE CAMPYLOBACTER CONUNDRUM

AMELIE GARENAUX,
CELINE LUCHETTI-MIGANEH,
GWENNOLA ERMEL,
FREDERIQUE BARLOY-HUBLER,
ROB DE JONGE, DIANE NEWELL,
SOPHIE PAYOT, MICHEL FEDERIGHI,
ODILE TRESSE, SANDRINE GUILLOU
AND MAGALI RITZ

Nova Science Publishers, Inc.
New York

Copyright © 2008 by Nova Science Publishers, Inc.

All rights reserved. No part of this book may be reproduced, stored in a retrieval system or transmitted in any form or by any means: electronic, electrostatic, magnetic, tape, mechanical photocopying, recording or otherwise without the written permission of the Publisher.

For permission to use material from this book please contact us:
Telephone 631-231-7269; Fax 631-231-8175
Web Site: http://www.novapublishers.com

NOTICE TO THE READER

The Publisher has taken reasonable care in the preparation of this book, but makes no expressed or implied warranty of any kind and assumes no responsibility for any errors or omissions. No liability is assumed for incidental or consequential damages in connection with or arising out of information contained in this book. The Publisher shall not be liable for any special, consequential, or exemplary damages resulting, in whole or in part, from the readers' use of, or reliance upon, this material.

Independent verification should be sought for any data, advice or recommendations contained in this book. In addition, no responsibility is assumed by the publisher for any injury and/or damage to persons or property arising from any methods, products, instructions, ideas or otherwise contained in this publication.

This publication is designed to provide accurate and authoritative information with regard to the subject matter covered herein. It is sold with the clear understanding that the Publisher is not engaged in rendering legal or any other professional services. If legal or any other expert assistance is required, the services of a competent person should be sought. FROM A DECLARATION OF PARTICIPANTS JOINTLY ADOPTED BY A COMMITTEE OF THE AMERICAN BAR ASSOCIATION AND A COMMITTEE OF PUBLISHERS.

Library of Congress Cataloging-in-Publication Data

Better understanding the Campylobacter conundrum / Amélie Garénaux ... [et al.].
   p. ; cm.
 Includes bibliographical references and index.
 ISBN 978-1-60456-636-9 (softcover)
 1. Campylobacter infections. 2. Campylobacter jejuni. I. Garénaux, Amélie.
 [DNLM: 1. Campylobacter jejuni--genetics. 2. Adaptation, Physiological. 3. Campylobacter Infections--microbiology. 4. Food Microbiology. QW 154 B565 2008]
 QR201.C25B48 2008
 664.001'579--dc22
                        2008015179

Published by Nova Science Publishers, Inc. ✢ *New York*

Contents

Preface		vii
Chapter I	General Introduction	1
Chapter II	Campylobacter jejuni and Food Safety	3
Chapter III	Campylobacter Genomes: General and Specific Features	27
Chapter IV	From Environment to the Host: Stress Resistance Mechanisms and Regulation Pathways	39
Chapter V	Other Strategies Developed by Campylobacter to Adapt to the Environment	67
Chapter VI	General Conclusion	93
References		95
Index		135

Preface

Campylobacter jejuni is a microaerophilic and thermophilic pathogen genetically close to *Helicobacter pylori*. It represents one of the most important emerging food pathogens, as it is one of major sources of human enteritis, in developed as well as in developing countries. It is also a source of rare, but serious, neuropathies. The interest in this bacterium has constantly been growing during the last two decades, and is enhanced because of emerging antibiotic resistant strains. The sequencing of the *C. jejuni* genome has revealed a small genome in which a lot of those regulation systems, fully understood in well-studied bacteria, are absent. To infect humans, a pathogen has to survive different environmental stresses and attacks of the immune system, and also be able to express its virulence factors. The *Campylobacter* conundrum is: how does this microaerophilic (sensitive to oxygen) bacterium, owning a small genome and lacking most of the well-known regulation systems, still constitute a hazard for humans? From what is known about the *C. jejuni* genome, this review proposes to draw a parallel between, on the one hand the different mechanisms and regulation pathways existing, and on the other hand stress resistance and virulence of this emerging food pathogen.

Chapter I

General Introduction

Campylobacter jejuni is a spiral-shaped microaerophilic bacterium causing gastro-enteritis in humans. The symptoms of campylobacteriosis are severe abdominal pain and acute diarrhea. In some rare cases, *Campylobacter* infection can result in postinfectious complications like arthritis or neuropathologies, such as Guillain-Barre syndrome [9]. Public health authorities throughout the world are acting to identify, quantify and limit food poisoning caused by these microorganisms. Surveillance programs allow estimation of the risk, but adopted measures can only be determined from a detailed knowledge of (1) the sources of contamination, (2) the contamination levels, (3) the different environmental conditions encountered from the natural source to the human host and their impact at the cell, as well as at the population, level, and (4) the virulence factors and the conditions affecting their expression. Three complete genome sequences of *C. jejuni* are now available [113, 159, 294] (and more are in progress) but even though major advances have been made in the understanding the environmental stress resistance mechanisms and pathogenicity of *C. jejuni*, it is still unclear how this microorganism, sensitive to oxygen and growing at high temperatures, survives in the environment and represents today one of the major causes of food poisoning in industrialized as well as in developing countries. This observation is often referred to as the "*Campylobacter* conundrum" [175]. New insights, brought by analysis of the complete genome sequences, recently became available and studies on environmental stress resistance mechanisms show that although *C. jejuni* possesses a small genome with few of the known general regulation pathways, a broad range of adaptations are induced under unfavourable conditions to allow the bacterium to reach its human host, survive in the intestinal tract and express its virulence factors. As they constitutes an interface between the pathogen and its host or environment, particular focus will be given to *C. jejuni* membranes and how they are used for protection, to detect environmental change, to exchange metabolites or to allow the contact of virulence factors with human cells.

Chapter II

Campylobacter jejuni and Food Safety

1.1. A Microaerophilic and Thermotolerant Pathogen (General, Phenotype and Physiology)

1.1.1. History and Taxonomy

Today known as one of the principal causes of food poisoning in industrialized countries, historically *Campylobacter* were first associated with animal health problems. Thus, from the first description of these germs in the stools of diarrheic children by Escherichia in 1886 in Germany and their first isolation by McFadyean and Stockman in 1913 [242], up until the middle of the 1940's, spiral bacteria called "vibrions" were regularly identified in association with problems of abortion or episodes of diarrhea in ovines, bovines and porcines. These microorganisms differed from true vibrions by their microaerophilic character and were named *Vibrio fetus* for those isolated from abortions, or *Vibrio jejuni* and *Vibrio coli* for those isolated from feces. The probable implication of these microbes in infectious disease of food origin was established in 1946 when Levy described a gastroenteritis epidemic in a prison population in Illinois in the United States [213]. He reported that microorganisms resembling *Vibrio jejuni* had been found in 13 blood cultures from patients, in 20 % of fecal samples and in the milk distributed to the prisoners. This was probably the first description of digestive campylobacteriosis of food origin.

Until 1963 these microaerophilic vibrions were included in the *Vibrio* genus. At this time, Sebald and Veron proposed the creation of the *Campylobacter* genus (etymologically from the Greek kampulos = curved, bacter = rod) [341], with a species type *Campylobacter fetus*. Since then, the upsurge in taxonomy has enabled the establishment of the classification of these microorganisms. *Campylobacter*, along with *Arcobacter* and *Sulfurospirillum*, belong to the family of *Campylobacteraceae*, from the *Campylobacterales* order (with *Helicobacteraceae* and *Hydrogenimonadaceae* families), in the *Epsilonproteobacteria* class of the *Proteobacteria phylum*, in the *Eubacteria* domain.

Table 1. Genus *Campylobacter*: species and sub-species

Species	Sub-species
Campylobacter coli	
Campylobacter concisus	
Campylobacter curvus	
Campylobacter fetus	C. fetus subsp. venerealis
	C. fetus subsp. fetus
Campylobacter gracilis	
Campylobacter helveticus	
Campylobacter hominis	
Campylobacter hyointestinalis	C. hyointestinalis subsp. hyointestinalis
	C. hyointestinalis subsp. lawsonii
Campylobacter insulaenigrae	
Campylobacter jejuni	C. jejuni subsp. doylei
	C. jejuni subsp. jejuni
Campylobacter lanienae	
Campylobacter lari	
Campylobacter mucosalis	
Campylobacter rectus	
Campylobacter showae	
Campylobacter sputorum	C. sputorum biovar Sputorum
	C. sputorum biovar Fecalis
	C. sputorum biovar Paraureolyticus
Campylobacter upsaliensis	

To date, the genus *Campylobacter* includes a variety of very heterogeneous species having highly diverse habitats, such as the buccal cavity of man (*C. concisus, C. curvus* and *C. showae*), the preputial cavity of bulls (*C. fetus* subsp. *venerealis* and *C. sputorum* subsp. *bubulus*) or the digestive tube of warm-blooded animals (*C. jejuni, C. coli* and *C. lari*) (Table 1). Among these species one is largely predominant over the others in its involvement in problems related to the safety of foodstuffs: *Campylobacter jejuni*. One should note, however, that despite this predominance, other species are of interest in food hygiene, principally *C. fetus* subsp. *fetus, C. coli, C. upsaliensis* and *C. lari*. In addition, authors rarely distinguish between *C. jejuni* subsp. *doylei* and *C. jejuni* subsp. *jejuni* on account of the difficulty of diagnosis (absence of growth of *C. jejuni* subsp. *doylei* at 42°C among other factors). Hence the term *C. jejuni* generally refers to *C. jejuni* subsp. *jejuni* and this will be the case in the remainder of this chapter.

1.1.2. Bacteriology

Campylobacter jejuni is a Gram-negative bacillus, fine and curved, 0.2 to 0.5 microns in diameter and 1 to 8 microns long, in the shape of a comma, an "S", a helix or a spiral. It displays one or several waves and usually has a single polar flagellum, although a flagellum at each pole has been described in stages of pre-division. This structure gives the microorganism great mobility, easily observed under the microscope, which is much used for its identification and as a diagnostic tool. *Campylobacter jejuni* is asporulate (nonsporeforming) and sometimes capsulated. After several days of culture, rounded or coccoid forms (0.5 microns in diameter) weaklier staining often appear. It would seem that these may be equivalent to degenerate forms, even if such coccoid cells have sometimes been implicated in the concept of viable but nonculturable forms (VBNC, see §3.1).

Campylobacter jejuni is considered to be a microaerophilic bacterium, *i.e.* grow in the presence of an atmosphere poor in oxygen, generally between 5 and 10 %. In an ambient atmosphere, accumulation of peroxides in the cell inhibits its growth (see §3.2). To achieve an optimal yield, the culture media should contain compounds, which trap toxic elements and/or favour the synthesis by *C. jejuni* of detoxifying enzymes (sodium pyruvate, thioglycolate, ferrous sulfate, blood, charcoal....).

Many authors find that *Campylobacter jejuni* is more capnophilic than microaerophilic, *i.e.* that it requires an atmosphere enriched in CO_2 to proliferate (generally 10 %). Most often, but not exclusively, the gaseous mixture appropriate for culture of the microbe is: $O_2 = 5$ %; $CO_2 = 10$ %; $N_2 = 85$ %.

All species of the *Campylobacter* genus can proliferate at 37°C and are true mesophiles. *C. jejuni* grows at temperatures ranging from 30 to 45 °C and its optimal pH zone is from 6.5 to 7.5. Finally, the presence of 0.5 % sodium chloride (NaCl) in the medium is recommended for culture, whereas concentrations exceeding 1.5 % tend to inhibit growth. In broth, culture in planktonic suspension is visible as a faint cloudiness, more apparent in the upper part of the tube just underneath the surface. In Petri dishes the colonies usually appear after 24 to 48 hours and are of the following types:

- S (Smooth). These are round, elevated and convex, of small diameter (1 - 2 mm), smooth and shiny with a regular border and at maturity display metallic reflections.
- R (Rough). These are spread out, flat and grey, sometimes granulose and transparent with an irregular border.
- CG (Cut Glass). Small (1 mm in diameter), round, elevated and translucent, these colonies refract the light in a mosaic of reflecting facets.

Table 2. Summary of growth conditions for *Campylobacter jejuni*

	OPTIMA	INHIBITION
Temperature	37 to 41,5°C	< 30°C or >45°C
pH	6,5 - 7,5	< 4,7 or >8,2
O_2	5 - 10%	0% or > 15-19%
CO_2	10%	-
a_w	0,997	< 0,987
NaCl	0,5%	1,5%

1.1.3. Typing

1.1.3.1. Biotyping

Several biochemical properties specific to *Campylobacter* are known today and some of them are of taxonomic and diagnostic interest.

The main biochemical characteristics of *Campylobacter jejuni* are:

- Oxidase +.
- Catalase +.

- Nitrate +.
- Glucides are neither oxidized nor fermented in Hugh and Leifson's medium.
- The Voges-Proskauer reaction is negative (VP-).
- The methyl red reaction is negative (MR-).
- Indoxyl acetate hydrolysis +.
- Selenite reduction negative.
- Urease negative.
- Hydrogen sulfide (H_2S) production is negative in triple sugar iron medium.
- Generally, hippurate hydrolysis +.

This list is obviously not exhaustive since other biochemical properties exist and such properties have been used to develop diverse biotyping systems. Many authors have combined several characteristics in different ways, thereby proposing numerous biotyping schemes, but without any one scheme emerging as a reference. These systems have been exploited in epidemiological studies carried out on large numbers of strains. However, the extraordinary variety of responses obtained for the strains of a single species and the absence of correlation with other typing methods (see below) have made biotyping obsolete and less and less used today. Apart from the fact that these methods are time consuming, certain tests are difficult to perform and/or interpret.

1.1.3.2. Serotyping

Various antigen types have been described in *Campylobacter* and they may be reasonably divided into:

- Thermolabile antigens: corresponding roughly to proteins of the external membrane, flagellum (AgH) or capsule (AgK); these antigens are in general strongly immunogenic and widely used for serological typing.
- Thermostable antigens: these may be assimilated to somatic antigens of a lipopolysaccharide nature (LPS/AgO) but likewise include certain components of the cytoplasm and proteins of the external membrane.

To carry out antigenic identification of a pure strain, the currently recognized typing systems have to be followed, namely:

- Penner's scheme (1983) based on the use of thermostable antigens (essentially LPS) [300].
- Lior's scheme (1982) which employs thermolabile protein antigens [220].

1.1.3.3. Phagetyping

The determination of lysotype is an identification technique based on selective lysis by bacteriophages. The first lytic phage was described in *Campylobacter fetus* in 1970.

Grajewski *et al.* (1985) developed a standardized lysotyping technique to study the epidemiology of human infections caused by *C. jejuni* and *C. coli* [130] and this scheme has since been regularly improved and extended. Lior reported in 1989 the characterization of 38 lysotypes of *C. jejuni*, the most frequent in strains of human origin being the lysotypes 11.3 and 10. These results were confirmed in 1992 by Khakhria and Lior [192], who succeeded in classifying 80 % of 754 strains of *Campylobacter* (672 *jejuni* and 82 *coli*) in 46 different lysotypes. The typing scheme used at the time did not allow the lysotyping of other *Campylobacter* species (68 strains tested).

Another lysotyping system proposed by Salama *et al.* (1990) allowed discrimination of 140 different lysotypes among *C. jejuni* and *C. coli* species with the aid of 10 new phages added to Grajewski's scheme [333]. In epidemiological studies, lysotyping gives more precise information on strain origin than serotyping and seems in any case to be more reliable, being less subject to antigenic variations. Thus, in a collection of 754 strains of *C. jejuni* isolated from sporadic human cases of campylobacteriosis, Wareing *et al.* (2002) distinguished 33 and 42 different subtypes using Penner's serotyping and Salama's lysotyping scheme, respectively [399]. Applying Preston's biotyping system to the same collection, Bolton *et al.* (1992) had obtained 106 different subtypes [41]. One should further note that in many studies some strains remained nontypable by these methods.

1.1.3.4. Molecular Typing

The techniques described above are rarely used today and have been supplanted by methods based on analysis of DNA polymorphism. In fact, typing of strains by PCR-RFLP (Restriction Fragment Length Polymorphism), RAPD

(Random Amplified Polymorphism DNA) or PFGE (Pulsed Field Gel Electrophoresis) allows further discimination and the tracing of sources and routes of contamination (see below). Dingle *et al.* (2001) proposed a protocol for the application of MLST (MultiLocus Sequence Typing) to *C. jejuni* [91]. This method enables precise analysis of the genetics of populations and their evolution. It is based on amplification and sequencing of several regions of the genome corresponding to genes coding for enzymes of intermediate metabolism, the so-called "housekeeping genes". The various strains tested are then differentiated by study of the different alleles they carry. The sensitivity and portability of this technique make it a potential tool for the identification of contamination sources. A specialized database is available on the Internet for centralization of results and global analysis of the population. It was however demonstrated by Sails *et al.* (2003) that although MLST presents several advantages (reproducibility, standardization, contribution to the centralization of data), it has to be coupled to another method to achieve a level of discrimination equivalent to that of PFGE [331].

1.1.4. Campylobacter Jejuni in Humans

1.1.4.1. Transmission to Man

Two principal modes of transmission of *Campylobacter* have been identified, namely direct and indirect. Transmission through direct contact with a reservoir is a relatively rare event affecting mainly farmers, veterinarians and abattoir workers (cases of occupationally-acquired illness). Nevertheless, transmission through contact with household pets, contaminated bathing waters or (rarely) a patient excreting bacteria should not be neglected. Indirect transmission usually involves a food vector and this mode is responsible for at least 80 % of campylobacteriosis cases [11]. It is difficult to estimate the relative importance of the food sources due to the small proportion of epidemic cases among all known cases of campylobacteriosis. The notifications are mostly sporadic and it is not easy to distinguish tendencies. The minimal dose causing infection has been estimated to a few hundreds of cells in milk [34]. On the other hand, case control studies have repeatedly highlighted the role of chicken meat (Table 3). This was supported by a survey performed in Belgium during the dioxin crisis, which showed that the number of campylobacteriosis cases had diminished by 40 % over the period of withdrawal of poultry from the market [391].

Table 3. Main risk factors associated with *Campylobacter* enteritis in twelve case-control studies

Country	Number of cases	Number of controls	Main risk factors	Ref.
USA (Washington)	218	526	Consumption of undercooked chicken, raw fish and shellfish	[143]
USA	45	45	Consumption of chicken. Contact with a cat	[87]
Norway	52	103	Consumption of chicken bought raw and sausages cooked on a barbecue	[181]
New Zealand	100	100	Consumption of chicken outside the home and untreated water	[165]
Switzerland	167	282	Overseas travel. Consumption of chicken	[338]
United Kingdom	598	598	Handling of raw meat. Contact with a diarrheic pet. Consumption of untreated water	[3]
New Zealand	621	621	Consumption of chicken undercooked or in a restaurant. Overseas travel. Use of rainwater. Consumption of raw milk. Contact with animals	[100]
Sweden	101	198	Consumption of raw milk. Consumption of chicken and pork. Food cooked on a barbecue	[364]
USA (Hawaii)	211	211	Consumption of chicken outside the home. Ingestion of antibiotics	[101]
Denmark	282	319	Consumption of undercooked chicken, red meat cooked on a barbecue, grapes and raw milk. Overseas travel	[269]
Norway	212	422	Consumption of untreated water, meat cooked on a barbecue and chicken bought raw. Contact with animals. Consumption of undercooked pork	[182]
USA	1316	1316	Consumption of chicken outside the home and red meat prepared in a restaurant. Contact with animal feces or young pets	[118]

1.1.4.2. Foodborne Diseases

In the United States, the annual number of infections with *Campylobacter* is estimated to be 2.1 to 2.4 million, which is greater than the number of salmonelloses [117]. The incidence of confirmed campylobacteriosis was estimated by the foodnet system to 12.72/100,000 inhabitants in 2005 [253]. In Europe (25 countries), a total of 183,961 confirmed cases of campylobacteriosis were recorded in 2004, the mean incidence for all countries being 47.6/100,000 inhabitants. On both continents, *Campylobacter jejuni* was the dominant species (81 to 94 % of cases) in *Campylobacter* infections. These data confirm that today this microorganism is the most commonly reported gastrointestinal bacterial pathogen in humans in industrialized countries.

1.1.5. How Can We Control *Campylobacter jejuni* in Food Industry?

Control of animal reservoirs and hence reduction of the selection pressure is an important strategy which must be reinforced. This aspect will be developed in the next chapter (see below).

There exist two principal approaches to control *Campylobacter jejuni* in processed foodstuffs:

- prevention of contamination in food industry, during transport and in food preparation inside or outside home;
- total or partial elimination of *Campylobacter jejuni* from foods by physical or chemical methods.

1.1.5.1. Prevention of Contamination

The sources of *Campylobacter* contamination are numerous and it is therefore essential to control all possible entry points of bacteria, from the site of livestock breeding or water treatment, to the consumer.

To avoid any proliferation in water supply networks, installations must be both well designed and well maintained. Water treatment must be suitable for this type of contamination and its efficacy should be tested regularly.

The animal and notably the avian reservoir being the principal source of contamination, measures must be taken right from breeding to prevent colonization (see §1.2). Specific measures for abattoirs defined during the development of HACCP (Hazard Analysis Critical Control Point) initiatives advocate the control testing of raw materials and the avoidance of mixing of different batches. The equipment and working areas must be regularly disinfected and the maintenance of the machines carried out regularly. It is also important to ensure that the different scalding and chilling protocols are strictly respected. All along the production chain, the personnel must respect the hygiene regulations and systematically eliminate carcasses, which do not conform.

The transporters and distributors must take care to employ the correct storage conditions and to never put raw meat with other non-contaminated produce. If this is necessary, it is strongly recommended to use protective films.

Finally, the ultimate precautions concern the consumer. It is essential to clean the refrigerator regularly and to carefully separate raw meat from other food. The tools used to cut up meat should be systematically washed before any other use. One should avoid drinking raw milk or untreated water and ensure that meat is thoroughly cooked (one can for example cook or pre-cook meat before putting it on the barbecue). A study of cross contamination in kitchens found it advisable to reserve certain working areas specifically for poultry and recommended improving the level of hygiene in family kitchens [201].

1.1.5.2. Survival and Destruction of Bacteria in Food

The treatments undergone during the processing, transport and distribution of food, as likewise the bacteriological characteristics of *Campylobacter,* do not favor the proliferation of this microorganism in the finished product. Hence in the absence of recontamination the risk of infection does not increase. One even generally observes a decrease in the number of bacteria. However, the survival can be more or less important depending on the treatments and also on the bacterial strains, which display variable resistance to the different stresses undergone.

Physical Treatment

Heat and Cold

At temperatures of freezing (-20°C) and refrigeration (0 to 10°C) the survival remains significant. A study performed on chicken showed that refrigeration at 4°C led to a reduction of the population of 0.31 to 0.81 $\log_{10}$ CFU/g in 3 to 7 days and freezing to a reduction of 0.56 to 3.39 $\log_{10}$ CFU/g in 2 weeks [33]. During these forms of treatment, increasing the air speed diminished survival in the product while increasing its desiccation, although the texture of chicken skin seemed to protect the bacteria from this effect.

Campylobacter are on the other hand very sensitive to high temperatures. Whatever the size of the population or the nature of the food matrix (liquid or solid), heating the entire sample to temperatures of over 60°C destroyed all the cells present within a few minutes (table 4).

Table 4. D values of *Campylobacter jejuni* for some media and foods [110]

Liquid media			
	Heating (°C)	D value (min)	Nb of tested strains
Phosphate buffer	58	0.24 – 0.28	3
Milk	53	1 – 2.2	3
	56	0.3 – 0.9	2
	60	0.2 – 0.3	3
Solid media			
	Heating (°C)	D value (min)	
Poultry	50	8,7 – 9,2	5
	55	2,12 – 2,25	5
	58	0,7 – 0,9	5
Red meat	60	0,2 – 0,34	8

Irradiation

Campylobacter are also highly sensitive to ionizing radiation. The irradiation parameters necessary for their inactivation are largely inferior to those required to eliminate other enteropathogens like salmonella or *E. coli*. Thus, doses of less than or equal to 1 kGy are quite sufficient to significantly reduce the number of viable cells and may be recommended to prevent infection by *Campylobacter* [214].

Table 5. D values (kGy) at different temperatures for a strain of *C. jejuni* treated in red meat [203]

Temperature	- 30°C	0°C	+ 30°C
D value	0,293 kGy	0,186 kGy	0,162 kGy

Ultraviolet Radiation

Use of U.V. lamps for germicide applications in the purification of water has been known for a long time. In 1987 Butler *et al.* investigated the sensitivity of *C. jejuni* to U.V. radiation at 254 nm [54]. This microbe appeared to be much more sensitive to ultraviolet radiation as compared to *E. coli* (1.8 versus 5 mws/cm^2) and they concluded that commercially available U.V. lamps could easily inactivate *C. jejuni*.

Microwaves

Choi *et al.* (1993) studied the survival of *C. jejuni* in milk after microwave treatment (1380 watts) [72]. Three minutes of heating (temperature reached 71.1°C) were sufficient to definitively eliminate all *C. jejuni* cells, whereas eight minutes were required for *Yersinia enterocolitica*. One minute of heating reduced the population of *C. jejuni* by more than 5 logs.

High Hydrostatic Pressure

Some recent but still rare studies have clearly shown that treatments of relatively short duration (10 min) at pressures of less than 400 MPa are sufficient to obtain an important decimal reduction of the population, the effect increasing with increasing pressure [349]. As in the case of other physical methods, a protective role of the food with respect to the treatment has been demonstrated, as compared to treatment in artificial media (buffers or broths) [240].

Chemical Treatment or Modification of the Atmosphere

The pH of most products susceptible to harbor *Campylobacter* is compatible with survival of the microbe, whereas it survives poorly when the pH lies below 4 or above 9. The foods and drinks most frequently incriminated in cases of campylobacteriosis (meat, milk, water) thus have a pH compatible with survival of the bacteria. On the contrary, an important bacteriostatic effect is observed at pH values of less than 4, particularly when the drop in pH is due to the presence of organic acids. Salting or addition of ascorbic acid likewise diminishes the survival of *Campylobacter*. Purification of water by treatment with chlorine enables rapid destruction of a *Campylobacter* contamination. Chlorine is also used in the United States to clean carcasses and thereby permits partial reduction of the population (0.5 $\log_{10}$ CFU/ml after cleaning with water containing 25-35 ppm chlorine) [26]. Similarly, cleaning of carcasses by passage through a bath containing trisodium phosphate results in an important decrease in the level of contamination (by about 2 logs).

Addition of ascorbic acid to a nutritive medium (5 mmol/L) has a bactericidal effect on *C. jejuni* at 42°C and according to the work of Juven *et al.* (1988) [178], this effect would appear to extend to meat. These authors inoculated two batches of turkey meat with *C. jejuni* and stored them at +5°C for 7 weeks. As of the second week, the samples supplemented with 5-mmol/kg ascorbic acid gave a culturable cell count 2 logs lower than that of non-supplemented control samples.

The survival of *Campylobacter* is limited in an atmosphere enriched in O_2. Conversely, the conditioning of food products under vacuum or in an atmosphere enriched in CO_2 does not seem to lead to any notable decrease in the survival of the bacteria [98].

Table 6. D values (days) of *C. jejuni* in Brucella broth for different atmospheres at 4 or 25°C

Atmosphere	D value (days)			
	100% N2	5% O2 + 10% CO2 + 85% N2	Air	100% O2
4°C	8,71 (± 0,52)	6,17 (±1,41)	2,88 (±0,5)	2,09 (± 0,84)
25°C	1,34 (±0,9)	1,25 (±0,04)	1,03 (± 0,09)	0,77 (±0,29)

Miscellaneous

Bacteriocins

In 1992 Schoeni and Doyle isolated bacteria colonizing the cecum of white leghorn laying hens free of *C. jejuni* [337]. Nine strains were found to produce metabolites against *Campylobacter* (colicins). More recently, Stern *et al.* (2006) demonstrated the efficacy of a bacteriocin produced by a strain of *Lactobacillus salivarius* in reducing the carriage of *Campylobacter* by chickens [360].

The Lactoperoxidase System

Beumer *et al.* (1985) were the first to reveal the bactericidal action of the lactoperoxidase system of raw milk on *C. jejuni* [32] . This enzyme system leads to a rapid decrease in the number of culturable cells in raw milk. In the same manner, addition of lactoperoxidase to artificially contaminated sterilized milk strongly reduces the number of culturable cells of *C. jejuni*. The lactoperoxidase system can however be readily inactivated by pasteurization.

Spices, Essential Oils and Tea

The effects of oregano, sage and cloves on *C. jejuni* have been studied at different temperatures. Globally, these three substances at concentrations of 0.5 % have an inhibitory action on *C. jejuni* during the first 16 hours of conservation. Fischer and Phillips (2006) recently demonstrated the efficacy of the essential oil of bergamot in significantly reducing populations of *E. coli* O157 and *C. jejuni* [111]. In this study the Gram-positive bacteria tested appeared to be more sensitive than the Gram-negative bacteria.

Diker *et al.* (1991) used gel diffusion to test the bactericidal effect of an extract of tea on *C. jejuni* [90]. The zone of inhibition of *C. jejuni* was largely superior to that of *Staphylococcus aureus*, whereas *E. coli* were not inhibited. The molecule or molecules responsible for this bactericidal property were not of a proteic nature.

Trisodium Phosphate

TSP (trisodium phosphate) is employed in the USA to reduce numbers of *Campylobacter* and other contaminants present on poultry carcasses. In this country, the treatment is generally carried out after refrigeration by plunging the carcasses in a bath of 10 % TSP at 50°C for 15 s [346]. This procedure decreases the mean level of contamination of the poultry by 1.2-1.5 logs. In France, Federighi *et al.* (1995) obtained a reduction of 1.3 logs in the mean level of contamination of chicken carcasses by thermotolerant *Campylobacter*, the treatment being performed after evisceration [108].

Disinfectants

Campylobacter do not seem to display any particular resistance to the disinfectants commonly used in the food industry, although few investigations have been devoted to this subject. An *in vitro* study by Avrain *et al.* (2003) showed that treatment with benzalkonium chloride (1 %) or sodium hypochlorite (0.63 %) allowed easy elimination of several strains of *Campylobacter* [19].

Conclusion

Campylobacter jejuni represent today a major cause of food poisoning throughout the world. Asymptomatic intestinal carriage of these bacteria by domestic livestock makes the animal reservoir the principal source of contamination of food products and indeed throughout the human food chain. Nevertheless, the careful application of suitable measures of hygiene, from production to consumption, allows the reduction of risk of contamination of foodstuffs by *Campylobacter*. The survival capacities of this microorganism, for a long time underestimated, have now been reassessed in the light of new findings derived from genomic studies concerning the physiology of the microbe. This information confirms that a better knowledge of *Campylobacter* survival mechanisms and a detailed understanding of *Campylobacter* pathogenic potential are required. This will enable us to precisely evaluate the danger represented by this microorganism and, thus, to correctly assess *Campylobacter* risk management options.

1.2. Epidemiology of Thermophilic Campylobacters –Veterinary and Environmental Aspects

Introduction

The *Campylobacter* species *C. jejuni* and *C. coli* are remarkably successful organisms. They are detectable in a vast range of host species where they usually colonise the intestinal tract but can also be isolated from a range of other tissues, including spleen and liver, even in the absence of disease. The physiological properties of such campylobacters indicate that they can only grow in the host (or in a laboratory) but, nevertheless, they are ubiquitous in the environment and, recoverable from a variety of sources like water and soils where they successfully survive for long periods.

In this section, veterinary epidemiological aspects including the colonisation of domestic and wild animals and birds will be considered. In addition the survival of the organisms in the environment will be reviewed. Lastly the risks of these epidemiological factors to human health will be evaluated.

1.2.1. Domestic Livestock

A range of *Campylobacter* species, can be found colonising the gut and shed in the faeces of all domestic livestock including cattle, sheep, pigs. Of the thermophilic species these are primarily *C. jejuni*, *C. coli* and *C.hyointestinalis*, but *C. fetus* subsp. *fetus* a non-thermophilic species is also common. These gut infections are usually asymptomatic but in pregnant cattle and sheep all of these campylobacters can cause abortion or infertility. Most of these species can cause disease in humans, however, in this section mostly only *C. jejuni* and *C. coli* will be further considered.

The presence of *C. jejuni* and *C. coli* carriage in domestic livestock is common. The prevalence of infection has been investigated in many studies [271] but relatively few countries have undertaken surveys of national herds, which commands considerable resource. Denmark [14] routinely surveys cattle and pigs at slaughter for campylobacters and in 2005 found 42.5% and 85.4% to be positive, respectively. Similarly in a recent (2003) national survey of animals at slaughter in Great Britain [418] 54.6% of 667 cattle, 43.8% of 713 sheep and 69.3% of 528 pigs had recoverable campylobacters in their faecal/rectal samples. Because of the well-recognised fragility of campylobacters, the results of such surveys are highly dependant on the microbiological methodologies as well as the speed of transport to the laboratories [418]. Nevertheless, using similar methodologies some differences in prevalence between developing and industrialised countries has been noted [193].

Differences in culture methodology may also explain some of the variations in species detected among such animals. In the Great Britain survey [418] of cattle and sheep at slaughter, the species recovered were predominantly, but not solely, *C. jejuni* (81% and 65% respectively) while in Denmark only *C. jejuni* was recovered from cattle. Interestingly in a PCR-based study in Canada *C. lanienae* [166] was the predominant species identified but this has not been reported in culture-based surveys even though it is able to grow at 42°C.

Seasonality in prevalence of carriage in livestock is debatable. There is little evidence for seasonality in cattle at slaughter [418, 355] but carriage in dairy cows may have a seasonality with peaks in spring and autumn [355] perhaps associated with movement to and from grass and suggesting that campylobacter carriage can be affected by stress.

The numbers of organisms shed into the environment from livestock may be significant with between 6×10^2 and 3×10^4 quoted [355] though this is age dependant [276]. Many strain types are present in cattle but recent evidence suggests that some strains (*i.e.* ST-61) may be specifically adapted for the cattle gut [1, 31, 114].

The evidence suggests that Campylobacter carriage in bovines is age related. Infection in calves is acquired soon after birth [131] and in some cases could be caused by contaminated milk as a result of campylobacter mastitis [163]. Carriage reaches a peak in young animals and then declines [276]. This is reflected in, not only the prevalence of colonisation, but also the numbers of campylobacters excreted. This suggests that there is some limiting factor in carriage; possibly acquired immunity. Using molecular typing, sources of infection for cattle potentially include wild birds, rodents and flies [4] but interesting an increased prevalence of carriage in feedlot cattle over time from first entry, suggests horizontal transmission from other cattle is also important [31].

Little is known of the epidemiology of campylobacters in sheep though faecal shedding is reported to be seasonal and at levels of about 10^4 cfu per gram feaces [355]. In New Zealand it appears that older animals have a lower prevalence of carriage [23], once again indicating acquired immunity limits colonisation.

Carriage of campylobacters in swine is extremely common. In all studies *C. coli* is the predominant species identified in swine, which suggests that this species has evolved to preferentially colonise the pig gut and that the ecological conditions in the swine gut provide a unique environment. This is supported by the evidence that at least some isolates of *C jejuni* from swine appear to be genotypically different from those isolated from other hosts [233]. Piglets become colonised soon after birth, apparently acquiring this infection from their dams [10, 145] and colonisation is maintained by incoming strains from other sources during fattening.

1.2.2. Poultry

It is generally considered that *C. jejuni/coli* have evolved mechanisms to optimally colonise the avian gut [209], which has a core temperature of 42°C. Surveys indicate that all domestic fowl, including chicken, turkey, geese, duck and pigeon, and most wild birds, are susceptible to asymptomatic colonisation. Only in ostrich is there clear evidence of an association between colonisation and disease. About 90% of the strains isolated from chickens are *C. jejuni*; the remainder are *C. coli*. However, older flocks (*i.e.* laying hens) and turkeys may have higher levels of *C. coli*. Most information available is focussed on broiler chicken flocks as these are considered a major risk to human health (reviewed below). This information is extensive and several recent detailed reviews are recommended [95, 272, 392].

The prevalence of campylobacter positive flocks varies remarkably [271]. Few national surveys have been undertaken but those that have indicated that, at least in European countries, flock positivity varies between 10-95% and this variation appears to reflect geographical environmental differences (Nordic countries having fewer positive flocks), and has seasonal peaks (usually in the summer months). In addition flock positivity is dependant on levels of biosecurity and management practices, with organic and free range flocks more frequently colonised than conventionally-reared flocks [157].

As far as detectable, chicks appear to be hatched campylobacter-free even though campylobacter colonization of the oviduct can occur. Colonisation is then age-associated, with usually a 2-3 week lag before becoming detectable. This lag may reflect protective maternal antibodies in the chicks [330]. Once the first bird is infected then fecal-oral spread is rapid and 100% of the flock can become colonised within days. Low levels of colonisation in a flock therefore may indicate recently acquired infection and such a situation may occur more frequently as interventions to reduce colonisation become more effective. Over time colonisation can wain such that older flocks, for example laying hens, can have reduced in-flock prevalence. This suggests that acquired specific immunity [66] in chickens can be protective and provides some hope that vaccines could be effacious.

The campylobacters colonise the mucus mainly of the lower small intestine and caecum. The infective dose can be lower than 10 cfu but after only 2 days numbers of campylobacter in the caeca can reach 10^9 cfu/gm ceacal contents. Faecal shedding is constant once colonisation occurs and can be enhanced by the stresses of handling and transportation [358].

Reduction of the prevalence of campylobacter-positive flocks is now a major strategic aim for policy makers in several countries. To achieve this the sources of infection for poultry flocks need to be understood. Using a combination of epidemiological methods and molecular epidemiology these sources are beginning to be identified. Vertical transmission is now largely discounted, at least as a significant factor in flock colonisation. Horizontal transmission, particularly via the movement of farm staff, is generally accepted as the major route [272]. Major factors increasing the risk of infection to a conventionally-reared broiler flock include; the presence of rodents, wildlife and domestic pets; other domestic livestock in adjacent fields; standing water on the farm; inadequate cleaning and disinfection between flocks; unchlorinated drinking water; and thinning or partial depopulation.

There are a range of intervention measures that can be taken to reduce the prevalence of campylobacters in poultry flocks [5, 95, 272, 392]. It is generally considered that improved biosecurity by farmers, such as the appropriate use of biosecurity barriers and reduction of human traffic, adequate cleaning and disinfection of houses, provision of clean water, effective wild life and rodent control and remoteness from other animals, will reduce campylobacter colonisation of conventionally-reared poultry flocks. However, the increased environmental exposure of flocks to campylobacters during the peak season (summer) or in free-range/organic management systems, tend to overwhelm such biosecurity measures. Complementary strategies, at the farm level, to reduce flock susceptibility are also required. Fortunately the lag phase in colonisation provides a window of opportunity of about 2-3 weeks to implement such strategies. Several such intervention strategies have been proposed and are under investigation. These include vaccination [84], competitive exclusion [138], application of bacteriophages [221] or bactericins [359] and bird genetic selection [44]. Considerable more work is needed on such intervention strategies before they can be applied commercially. In particular, there is an urgent need to understand the multiple bacterial and host factors involved in colonisation of chickens. With the use of modern genetic tools and analysis, including colonisation models to test defined mutants, and the increased availability of campylobacter genome sequences, these factors are just beginning to be investigated.

1.2.3. Domestic Pets

Dogs and cats are frequently colonised with *C. jejuni*, but are also colonised with other *Campylobacter* species including *C. coli, C. lari, C. upsaliensis* and *C. helveticus*. Faecal shedding can occur asymptomatically throughout life but is highest in dogs [139] and cats below one year of age [29]. Prevalence of infection with *C. jejuni* may be as high as 80% in some adult dog populations [2] but appears to be transitory with repeated exposure to multiple strains [139]. Colonisation can also be associated with diarrhoea, particularly in younger animals (kittens and puppies) but whether these organisms are causative is debatable and campylobacteriosis in these animals is difficult to reproduce experimentally.

1.2.4. Wild and Exotic Animals or Birds

As previously mentioned *Campylobacter* species are ubiquitous in the environment so it is not surprising that most wild and game birds, rodents, other wild life and even marine mammals can carry these organisms in their small intestines. It seems likely that some *Campylobacter* species preferentially colonise some hosts but the enterozoonotic campylobacters are common commensals in many of the wild animal and wild bird hosts. *Campylobacter jejuni/coli* can also be recovered from insects especially in environments heavily contaminated with the faeces of colonised livestock, but given the physiology of these organisms it seems likely that these are just chance traffickers rather than colonised hosts.

Routine veterinary bacteriology laboratories, required to investigate cases of enteritis in wild and exotic animals or birds, often recover campylobacters from such faecal material. It is very unlikely that these agents are causative of the enteric disease and interpretation of any such isolation should be undertaken with care.

1.2.5. Survival in Environmental Waters and Soils

The physiological properties of *C. jejuni* and *C. coli* ensure that under natural conditions bacterial growth only occurs within a warm-blooded host. Faecal shedding ensures and enables transmission to the next host and molecular epidemiological methods [114] indicate that the zoonotic strains circulate through the environment between the domestic livestock and wild animal/bird populations. Thus survival of campylobacters in the environment is a critical point in the ecology of this infection [344]. In the environment the bacteria are exposed to a number of hazardous stresses including ultraviolet light; temperature, pH and osmolarity extremes; atmospheric oxygen; and nutrient deprivation. Campylobacters are recognised as remarkably fragile organisms in the laboratory but regardless they survive in the environment sufficiently to cause infection in the next host. This conundrum is central to understanding the risks to human health of environmental campylobacters. Nevertheless, the bacterial mechanism(s) of survival remain unclear. Those mechanisms currently identified are reviewed in Murphy *et al.* (2006) [265] and, at least at the genetic level, may be unlike other bacteria occupying similar ecological niches. It is, however, clear that campylobacters survive best in cool, dark and moist environments and that some campylobacter strains survive better than others.

Despite the evidence for survival recovery of campylobacters from environmental sources is difficult. Frequently, recovered organisms are not sustainable in the laboratory under normal cultural conditions. Survival in water is a particular capacity of campylobacters, which has been widely investigated. The evidence for viable but non-culturable (VNC) forms is highly debatable and may just reflect normal bacterial death-associated changes but there is increasing evidence that biofilm formation [212] is important and even that intracellular survival in aqueous protozoa [348] can enhance survivability of campylobacters.

1.2.6. Risks to Human Health

Campylobacteriosis is a major cause of human enteritis worldwide. Human to human transmission is rarely observed so the sources of infection are primarily, if not wholly, veterinary. However, the routes of transmission and the relative importance of the various potential animal sources are unclear. Source attribution for human campylobacteriosis has been confounded by the ubiquitous nature of the organism, the paucity of outbreaks and, most importantly, by the ineffectiveness to date of molecular epidemiological investigations. This latter factor, coupled with the restricted survival of the organism, has largely precluded the use of typing methods to track campylobacters from patients through the environment to source.

C. jejuni and, to a lesser extent, *C. coli* demonstrate significant variability in both phenotypic and genotypic properties. A wide range of typing methods have been applied to large numbers of isolates from humans and animals [401]. Initially phenotypic methods like serotyping and/or phage typing were applied but the majority of strains were represented in a relatively few types so discriminatory power was poor. More recently, genotypic methods, which investigate variation at the genomic level using methods like pulse field gel electrophoresis (PFGE) or restriction fragment polymorphism of polymerase chain reaction products (PCR-RFLP) of variable genes such as *flaA* (fla typing) have been applied. Such methods have good discriminatory power but, unfortunately, genetic instability in campylobacters limits the usefulness of such methods. This plasticity in the campylobacter genome results from genomic rearrangements, single point mutations and the uptake of foreign DNA by natural transformation. The consequence is that the campylobacter population is only weakly clonal. Moreover, not only does genetic instability events frequently occur but, because this seems to be a mechanism of survival, the occurrence of these events is enhanced by environmental stresses. Thus, although such genotypic methods have enabled epidemiological investigations over short distances and times, for example through the poultry farm or abattoir environment, the approach is not so successful over the longer times and geographical distances involved in human disease attribution studies. Most recently multilocus sequence typing (MLST) has been applied to comparison of the populations of campylobacters causing disease in humans and the strains found in various animals [91]. The method relies on variations in the sequences of certain bacterial house keeping genes to define population evolutionary trends. The results of this approach suggest some association of certain sequence types with some host species [92]. These studies are now beginning to indicate the overlap between strains from humans and those from poultry and cattle but infrequently from other potential sources such as contaminated sands. Such studies will undoubtedly contribute to understanding of the source attribution of human campylobacteriosis in the future.

It is generally assumed that campylobacteriosis is a foodborne disease and that the major source is the handling and/or consumption of raw or undercooked poultry meat. This assumption is largely based on the high prevalence of campylobacter-contaminated poultry meat. This is a consequence of the faecal contamination of the feathers and skin of live birds arriving at the abattoir and the spillage of bird intestinal contents during processing. Properly cooked chicken is no risk to human health but, during poultry preparation in both domestic and commercial kitchens, cross-contamination of other uncooked products can readily occur. In some surveys, for example in Wales in 2002 [248], over 70% of poultry products are contaminated at retail. Levels of such contamination can exceed 10^6 cfu per carcass. Although the infective dose of *C. jejuni* in humans is both strain and host dependant, as few as 10^3 cfu organism can cause disease [34]. Recently, quantitative models have been developed to assess the risk of campylobacteriosis from poultry meat. These models are now being used to estimate the effectiveness of possible interventions [322] and have indicated that a reduction in the average bacterial load on chicken carcasses by 10^2 could generate a 30 fold reduction in human disease. However, dependence on such strategies should be measured as reducing the prevalence of campylobacter-positive flocks does not necessarily reduce human disease.

Classical epidemiological investigations, such as case-control studies, indicate that, in addition to poultry consumption, there is a wide range of potential food sources of infection. Estimates suggest that only between 20-40% of human campylobacteriosis cases are caused by poultry (A. Havelaar personal communication). Food related causes of the remaining cases include exposure to faecally-contaminated red meats (beef, pork and lamb), especially offal, and unpasteurised milk. The preparation methods for red meats minimises the risk but milk is easily contaminated by faecal material and campylobacter-associated mastitis has been reported as a cause of outbreaks [163]. Drinking water faecally-contaminated, with the runoff from livestock or by water fowl, and for which chlorination treatment has been inadequate, can also cause major outbreaks [202]. Finally, direct contact with pets, livestock or wild life, or with their waste products, are also identified as sources of human infection [121]. The absence of appropriate methods for tracking campylobacters precludes prioritorising these risks but *in vitro* studies clearly indicate that campylobacters from sources other than poultry have the same capacity to colonise and cause disease in humans [210]. Recently, flies have been hypothesised as a vector, transmitting campylobacters from animal faeces to human food [275].

The development of antimicrobial resistance in campylobacters may further contribute to the risk to human health. Although most cases of human campylobacteriosis are self limiting, about 10% require some form of medical intervention and in some individuals, especially the young, elderly and immunocompromised, this may include the use of antimicrobials. The recommended antimicrobial treatment is erythromycin but over recent years the fluoroquinolones have become the drug of choice, at least for adults. Resistance in campylobacters to a number of antimicrobials, especially nalidixic acid and the fluoroquinolones, has increased worldwide [55]. This increase has been largely blamed on the use of similar veterinary antimicrobials in food animal production and especially the use of enrofloxacin in poultry and has lead to the ban of enrofloxacin use in poultry in the USA.

Chapter III

Campylobacter Genomes: General and Specific Features

Introduction

In the past few years, genomic sequences of several epsilon-proteobacterial species from the *Campylobacterales* order have become available, including the completely sequenced genomes of three strains of *Campylobacter jejuni* (NCTC 11168 [294], RM1221 [113], 81-176 [159]) and one of *Campylobacter fetus* (Table 7-A). In addition, in January 2007, one can identify at least 13 sequencing projects of *Campylobacter*, a very great majority realized by the TIGR (Table 7-B) and concerning several *Campylobacter* species (viz. *C. lari*, *C. coli*, *C. upsaliensis* and *C. fetus*) and strains. Most of these sequences are now at the assembly stage and sequence information will be soon available in the NCBI database. The availability of these sequences opens new perspectives for comparative genomic studies on epsilon-proteobacteria and possibly, will lead to the discovery of novel molecular characteristics useful for diagnostics.

Table 7. *Campylobacter* genome sequencing projects (updated in January 2007)

A- Complete						
Organism	GC%	Diseases	Size (Kb)	ORFs	Accession	Reference-Date
C. jejuni jejuni NCTC 11168	31	Dia	1641	1654	NC_0 02163	[294]
C. jejuni RM1221	30	Dia	1809	1884	NC_0 03912	[113]
C. fetus fetus 82-40	33	Bct/Inf/Spt/Mgt	1773	1719	NC_0 08599	Unpublished 2006
C. jejuni jejuni 81-176	30	Dia/Gst	1616	1706	NC_0 08787	[159]

B- Under progress						
Organism	GC %	Type	Diseases	Size	ORFs Nb	Sequencing Center
C. coli RM2228	31	Pathogen	Gst/Spt	1860 Kb	-	TIGR
C. concisus 13826	39	Pathogen	Gig/Prs/Prd/Gst	2111 Kb	2039	TIGR
C. curvus 525.92	44	Pathogen	Gst/Pdi	1968 Kb	1909	TIGR
C. fetus	40	Pathogen	Inf/Spt/Mgt/Gif	1500 Kb		IIB-UNSAM
C. fetus fetus 82-40	33	Pathogen	Bct/Inf/Spt/Mgt	1773 Kb	1719	TIGR
C. hominis ATCC BAA-381	-	Non-Pathogen	None	-	-	TIGR
C. jejuni doylei 269.97	30	Pathogen	Bct	1878 Kb	1986	TIGR
C. jejuni jejuni 260.94	30	Pathogen	(GBS ??)	1657 Kb	1716	TIGR
C jejuni jejuni 84-25	30	Pathogen	-	1671 Kb	1748	TIGR
C. jejuni jejuni CF93-6	30	Pathogen	-	1676 Kb	1757	TIGR
C. jejuni jejuni HB93-13	30	Pathogen	(GBS ??)	1710 Kb	1694	TIGR
C. lari RM2100	29	Pathogen	Gst/Bct/Dia	1562 Kb	-	TIGR
C. upsaliensis RM3195	34	Pathogen	Gst/Bct/Dia/Spt	1773 Kb	-	TIGR

Diseases abbrevation : Septicemia=Spt, Gingivitis=Gig, Periodontis=Prs, Periodontosis=Prd, Gastroenteritis=Gst, Periodontal infection=Pdi, Infertility=Inf, Meningitis=Mgt, Genital infection=Gif, Bacteremia=Bct, Diarrhea=Dia.

2.1. *Campylobacter jejuni* NCTC11168 Genome

Campylobacter jejuni NCTC11168 genome was the first finished and published in 2000 by the Sanger Centre [294]. It was produced using a whole genome shotgun approach using several 1.4-2.2 kb pUC18 libraries. The unique circular chromosome sequence was generated from 33,824 sequencing reads and has 1,641,481 base pairs (30.6% GC) predicted to encode 1,654 proteins and 54 stable RNA species. Of the 1,654 predicted coding sequences (CDS), at least 20 probably represent pseudogenes; the average gene length is 948 bp, and 94.3% of the genome codes for proteins, making it the densest bacterial genome sequenced to date. Functional information (predicted function or informative profiles) was deduced for 77.8% of the CDS, leaving 13.5% genes of unknown function and 8.7% of orphan genes.

The GC bias of the chromosome indicates that the origin of replication lies near the start of the *dnaA* gene. Two large regions contain lower GC content (ca 25 %) corresponding to the lipooligosaccharide (LOS, Cj1135 to Cj1148) and extracellular polysaccharide (EP, Cj1421 to Cj1442) biosynthesis clusters. Strand bias is also evident as 61.1% of the CDS are transcribed in the same direction as replication. Except for these two LOS and EP clusters, for the two ribosomal protein operons and for the flagellar modification genes, *C. jejuni* chromosome appears to be little organized into functional clusters. Although genes fall into long closed sets, generally they appear to be functionally unrelated. Nevertheless, the strand-specific gene grouping suggests existence of co-transcription processes. Such absence of functional operons is particularly remarkable for genes involved in amino-acid biosynthesis since, except for genes coding *his, leu* and *trp*, those coding for *aro, asp, dap, gln, gly, ilv, met, phe, pro, ser, thr* and *tyr* genes are scattered randomly throughout the genome.

One surprising feature of the *C. jejuni* genome is the almost complete lack of repetitive DNA sequences with only four repeated sequences within the entire genome comprising the three copies of the rRNA operon. Apart from Cj0752, which is similar to part of IS605 *tnpB* from *H. pylori*, there is no evidence of any functional inserted sequence (IS) elements, transposons, retrons or prophages in the genome.

Another striking finding in *C. jejuni* genome was the presence of hypervariable sequences composed of short homopolymeric runs of nucleotides, mainly length variable poly-GC tracts. Such variations are commonly associated with genes involved in the surface properties phase variation (antigenicity) and may be important in the survival strategy of *C jejuni*. These variations that occurred during replication process could be favored by the faint arsenal of DNA repair genes in *C. jejuni*, which lack direct repair genes (*ada, phr*), glycosylases (*tag, alkA, mutM* and *nfo)*, mismatch repair genes (*vsr, mutH, mutL* and *sbcB*) and the SOS response genes (*lexA, umuC* and *umuD)*.

C. jejuni and *H. pylori* are closely related by 16S rRNA phylogeny, share many biological properties and were previously classified within the *Campylobacter* genus. In spite of this close phylogenetic relationship, both genomes share only 55.4% of orthologs, mainly in housekeeping functions. Like *H. pylori*, *C. jejuni* genome contains only three predicted sigma factors (*rpoD, rpoN* and *fliA*) but appears to have a broader repertoire of two-component regulatory systems. In most functions related to survival, transmission and pathogenesis, the organisms have remarkably little in common. This indicates that an important selective pressure created two very specific pathogens appropriate to their niches. 28.0% of *C. jejuni* genes show closest similarity to *E. coli*, 27.0% to *B. subtilis*, 4.6% to *Archeoglobus fulgidus* and 2.1% to *Saccharomyces cerevisiae*.

C. jejuni NCTC 11168 genome was recently completely re-annotated [137] with 1450 of the original 1654 CDS updated, leading a modification of over 20% (300) of precited functions.

2.2. Comparison Between *C. jejuni* Strains NCTC 11168 And RM1221

Strain RM1221 was sequenced and compared to the referent NCTC 11168 strain [293, 370]. Both genomes are syntenic but that RM1221 chromosome is disrupted by four genomic islands referred to as *Campylobacter jejuni*-integrated elements (CJIEs) and smaller gene clusters. The first genomic island, CJIE1, located upstream of *argC*, is a *Campylobacter* Mu-like phage encoding proteins [260]. CJIE2 and CJIE4 have several genes predicted to encode phage-related endonucleases, methylases, or repressors and are integrated into the 3' end of arginyl- and methionyl-tRNA genes, respectively. CJIE3 (integrated into the 3' end of an arginyl-tRNA) looks like an integrated plasmid, based on the observation that 73% of its predicted proteins show sequence similarity to *Campylobacter coli* RM2228 megaplasmid [113] and other *Campylobacter* plasmids [28, 279]. Also, 23% of CJIE3 products are similar to proteins found within the 71-kb pathogenicity island of *Helicobacter hepaticus* (HHGI1) [113]. The three elements, CJIE2, CJIE3, and CJIE4, were discovered to be adjacent to tRNA genes, which is commonly observed for other pathogenic islands [161]. A comparative genomic analysis [370] conducted from 67 *C. jejuni* and 12 *C. coli* strains, using both PCR-based and DNA microarrays assays demonstrated that these four CJIEs were also present in other *Campylobacter*. However, several CDS present within these CJIEs were absent or highly divergent in 26 *C. jejuni* strains, demonstrating high variability within these regions. 55% of the *C. jejuni* strains examined were positive for at least one CJIEs and 27% were positive for two or more. Interestingly, 58% of *C. coli* strains were also positive for these elements, although they only possessed either CJIE1 or CJIE3. CJIE1- Mu-like element and CJIE3-plasmid like elements have variable genomic insertion points. This variability may increase the genomic diversity of *Campylobacter* and supports the model for bacteriophage genome dynamics, as originally proposed by Hendrix *et al.* [152].

2.3. *C. jejuni* 81-176 Genome Exhibits Unique Pathogenic Features

C. jejuni 81-176 chromosome and plasmids were subjected to a high-throughput nucleotide sequencing to identify the relevant unique genomic features of this strain. Two sequencing runs were performed, producing 43 contigs and 60,905,794 bp of sequence (34-fold coverage). Gaps located within the LOS (56 bp) and capsule loci (1,589 bp) were closed using published sequences. The almost closed genome thus obtained is 1,594,651 bp long, with only two remaining gaps within highly repetitive regions: 32 bp within the internal sequences of rRNA operon and 111 bp within the highly conserved Cj0794 gene of NCTC 11168 [159].

C. jejuni 81-176 carries two resident plasmids, pVir and pTet (see below). Nevertheless, its genome is slightly smaller than those of NCTC 11168 and RM1221 strains due to a reduced number of genes involved in capsule and flagella synthesis and to the absence of prophages as seen in RM1221. However, it exhibits vestigial integrated element such as a complete additional type I DNA restriction-modification system probably acquired horizontally. The genomic structure of *C. jejuni* 81-176 is syntenic with NCTC 11168, except some duplications, deletions or insertion of genomic islands of various sizes. As said previously, the two referent strains contains several hypervariable plasticity regions that occur in gene clusters encoding LOS and capsule biosynthesis, as well as glycosylation loci. As expected, such diversity was also detected in 81-176 but in these hypervariable regions, analysis revealed the absence of 51 genes in *C. jejuni* 81-176 compared to NCTC 11168 [159].

C. jejuni 81-176 contains 37 genes, absent from both reference strains, located in 11 regions throughout the chromosome and involved in colonization and virulence. As examples, *C. jejuni* 81-176 encodes additional respiratory functions which may contribute to its unique ability to efficiently colonize its hosts' intestine: an additional gene cluster that encodes predicted DMSO reductase components of *Wolinella succinogenes* (DmsABCD), proposed to be important for respiration under oxygen-restricted conditions. Another example of the expanded respiratory pathways of *C. jejuni* 81-176 is the additional cytochrome c biogenesis cluster of genes (*cytC*), similar to the *C. lari* one but which specificity is still unknown. Within the same genomic segment, there is a gene encoding a putative γ-glutamyltranspeptidase (Ggt), only present in 81-176 and required for *H. pylori* colonization in animal models [71, 243]. This enzyme belongs to the antioxidant glutathione pathway and therefore may contribute to counteract oxidative stress. The role of Ggt in the pathogenesis of *C. jejuni* 81-176 was tested using a *ggt*-mutant. The mutant strain showed no growth defect and was able to enter and survive within cultured intestinal epithelial cells. However, its ability to colonize mice is significantly reduced. These results indicate that at least one of the unique *ggt* of *C. jejuni* 81-176 gene contributes significantly to virulence. The potential contribution to virulence of other *C. jejuni* 81-176 unique genes was also evaluated using *dmsA* and *cytC* mutants. These mutant strains showed no growth alteration (10% CO_2 or anaerobic conditions) and were able to enter and survive within intestinal epithelial cells. However, after 3 weeks of infection, *dmsA* mutant CFU in the mice feces were significantly reduced. In contrast, *cytC* mutant strain showed no detectable colonization defect.

Genomes of *C. jejuni* NCTC 11168 and RM1221 contain a relatively large number of pseudogenes, resulting of frameshifts or of significant degeneration of the ORFs. Interestingly, several of these pseudogenes encode apparently functional proteins in *C. jejuni* 81-176 such as *glpT* (glycerol-3-phosphate transporter), whose gene appears disrupted in RM1221 but intact in 81-176. The resulting ability to take up glycerol-3-phosphate may confer significant metabolic advantages on this strain. Another case concerns the genes encoding potassium-transporting ATPase (*kdpABC*) that are apparently functional in *C. jejuni* 81-176 although they are pseudogenes in both reference strains. It is possible that the presence of this additional system may benefit the growth of *C. jejuni* 81-176 in phagocytic vacuole, where the potassium concentration may be low [393].

2.4. *Campylobacter* Genome Comparison through CGH Arrays

Using *Campylobacter* microarray comparative studies, Taboada *et al.* [370] defined 16 intraspecies hypervariable genomic regions including the lipooligosaccharide biosynthesis (LOS), capsular biosynthesis (CAP), flagellar modification (FM) and DNA restriction/modification (R/M) loci. Interestingly, comparing the genomes of both NCTC 11168 and RM1221 strains demonstrated that strain RM1221 possessed genes distinct from strain NCTC 11168 in 11 of these 16 variable regions and was highly divergent in 13 of the 16 variable regions. An additional 17th hypervariable region (Cj0258-Cj0263) was also identified [370].

Genes which are different and common between the ATCC 43431 and NCTC 11168 strains were also identified by whole genome microbial CGH comparison [303]. Overall, 88 ORFs (5.3% of all ORFs) were found to be absent with high certainty in ATCC 43431 (85 further confirmed by PCR), whereas previous study from Dorrell *et al.* [94], identified 117 genes absent in this strain. Many of these dispensable genes were found to co-localize in five major chromosomal regions, referred to as plasticity zones PZ1 to PZ5. These zones were previously as hypervariable plasticity regions among *C. jejuni* strains [94, 299] and include genes encoding proteins involved in sugar modification and transport (PZ3), lipooligosaccharide (LOS) biosynthesis (PZ4) and capsular polysaccharide locus (PZ5). The absence of some genes in PZ1 such as Cj0265c (putative cytochrome c-type heme-binding periplasmic protein) and Cj0624c (molybdenum-containing enzyme C) suggests that strain ATCC 43431 is unable to utilize these electron acceptors. This is in agreement with the absence of the molybdenum transporter genes *modABC* in PZ2.

C. jejuni ATCC 43431 unique DNA fragments yield 83,909 bp, corresponding to a total of 130 ORFs. The average GC content of these ORFs (26.2%) is lower than that of the NCTC 11168 one (30.6%), which suggests that many of ATCC 43431-specific genes have been acquired through horizontal gene transfer. BLAST searches allowed the assignment of potential biological roles to 66% of the unique ORFs, *i.e* 86 ORFs classified in eight functional categories: cell envelope and surface, DNA modification, chemotaxis, bacteriophage, transport, small-molecule metabolism, hypothetical and unknown proteins. The first two categories constitute the major functional groups. As described above, LOS and capsule cluster genes vary between ATCC 43431 and NCTC 11168 (regions PZ5 for the capsular polysaccharide locus and PZ4 for the LOS biosynthesis locus). The observed gene variability in the LOS biosynthesis locus is supported by the difference in LOS structure between the two *C. jejuni* strains [369].

Four unique ORFs are homolog to integrases commonly promoting the integration of transposons into the host genome. Remarkably, 36 unique ATCC 43431 DNA fragments showed high similarity with 28 proteins from *H. hepaticus* ATCC 51449, in particular with 16 of the 70 proteins belonging to a possible pathogenicity island (HH0233 to 302) [365]. *C. jejuni* ATCC 43431 also harbours several *H. hepaticus* orthologs that are also homologous to genes from the *Rhizobium leguminosarum Imp* locus, involved in the temperature-dependent secretion of proteins and influences the level of infection in plants [35]. In *H. hepaticus*, these genes are part of a pathogenicity island that has been shown to be required for the induction of liver disease [365]. The identification of these Imp-like proteins, together with the identification of a TraG-like protein suggests that *C. jejuni* ATCC 43431 might be able to produce a type IV secretion system.

2.5. *Campylobacter* Plasmids Genomes

Plasmids have been found in between 19 and 53% of *C. jejuni* strains [376] and many of these have been reported to be R plasmids, transmissible among *Campylobacter* spp. but not to *Escherichia coli* [374, 376]. The importance of these plasmids in *Campylobacter* pathogenicity is still unclear and re-evaluation of their role is necessary, mainly through sequences analysis.

2.5.1. «Virulence Plasmids»

pVir Plasmid

The circular pVir plasmid of *Campylobacter jejuni* strain 81-176 was determined to be 37,468 nucleotides in length [21]. 83% of the plasmid correspond to coding information, significantly lower than *C. jejuni* NCTC 11168 (94% coding density). All but two of the ORFs were transcribed in the clockwise direction on the DNA plus strand. The overall GC content of the plasmid was 26%, lower than other *C. jejuni* and *coli* plasmids, which have GC % from 30.6 to 33.5 [226, 294]. However, a small cryptic plasmid from *Campylobacter hyointestinalis* has a similarly low G+C content of 28.3% [402].

pVir contains two large noncoding regions, one of them with a very low G+C content (19.8%) suggested to be the putative origin of replication. A total of 35 ORFs encoded predicted proteins with no significant orthologs in the current sequence databases and which to date appear to be *C. jejuni* specific. In addition, eight proteins had existing orthologs (two in *C. jejuni* NCTC 11168 and six in *H. pylori*) whose functions are currently unknown. All these predicted ORFs had suitable ribosome-binding sites (RBS, consensus AAGGA-N7-initiation codon). Only two of the predicted ORFs possessed an alternative start codon. This frequency of AUG initiation codons (96.3%) is higher than that seen for the NCTC 11168 chromosome (86.2%). There are 16 putative proteins encoded by pVir that are smaller than 100 residues and a further 19 that are between 100 and 200 residues. This represents an above-average proportion of low-molecular-weight proteins. However, the sequence quality of pVir was very high, and suitable RBSs preceded all these small proteins. The biological significance of the coding capacity of pVir being biased toward low-molecular-weight proteins is unknown. There are seven clustered genes on pVir that encode homologs of type IV secretion proteins. The type IV secretion system encoded by pVir shows its greatest similarity to type IV secretion proteins found in *H. pylori*. Various mutational analysis were done and show the importance of, at least 16 genes in the invasion process. pVir alone is insufficient for invasion, and appears remarkably stable in 81-176 and unable to be to cured.

pCC31/pTet Plasmid

The sequence of pCC31 (44 707 bp) revealed 50 ORFs, 44 transcribed in clockwise orientation with respect to *tetO*. The pTet is only 1 % larger than pCC31 (45 205 bp) and carries 49 ORFs, 43 being clockwise [28]. The DNA of the two plasmids are 94.3% identical with ca. 90.0 % of coding sequence. G+C contents are quite similar, 29.8 % (pCC31) and 29.1 % (pTet), and only slightly lower than the *C. jejuni* genome one (30.6 %) [294]. Only one G+C rich region was identified which contained *tetO* (40.4 % GC), suggesting a horizontal transfer origin for this gene. The two plasmids differ in two regions: in the first one, pCC31 contains *cpp15* encoding a protein 64 % similar to a hypothetical protein from *H. pylori* 26695 and absent in pTet. In the second region, the gene *cpp21* encodes a protein 50 % similar to another hypothetical protein from *H. pylori* J99. Additionally, there is a small ORF designated gene *cpp48* on pCC31 (but not pTet) that encodes a predicted protein of 6 kDa that shows no significant homology to known proteins. There are 19 cases where the alleles have different predicted lengths in pCC31 and in pTet. Some genes have modified 3' ends where the reading frames and stop codon of one allele appear to have been shifted. As the function of these genes is unknown, we cannot predict which of the frame-shifted variants are pseudogenes. There are 10 genes in pTet and pCC31 that encode predicted proteins with homology to T4SS multicomponent complexes that can translocate proteins and/or nucleoprotein complexes between bacteria through the cell envelope. Both plasmids encode a VirB2 homologue which represents the first pilin gene identified in *Campylobacter* [294]. They also carry a homologue of the VirB2-associated gene VirB5,6,7,8,9 and 10 (predicted to form a channel in the cytoplasmic membrane) and of the three ATPases associated with T4SS, VirB11, D4 and B4. Both plasmids also encode a putative DNA nickase and a helicase (*cpp26*) involved in generating single strand DNA as well as a ssDNA-binding protein ssb1 that may coat the single-stranded DNA during transfer.

2.5.2. Cryptic Plasmids

Small cryptic *Campylobacter* plasmids genomes are also available. As an example, two cryptic plasmids from an agricultural isolate of *Campylobacter coli* were also sequenced: p3384, (3316 bp, 31.18% of GC) and p3386 (2426 bp, 26,22 % GC). Each plasmid carry three putative ORFs detected: Mob-like, repA-like and repB like in p3384 and two hypothetical protein and one Rep 3-like in p3386 [173]. Another small cryptic plasmid, pCJ419, identified in a human clinical isolate of C. *jejuni* was also sequenced [8]. pCJ419 is a circular molecule (4013 bp, of 27.1% of GC) with a 22 bp AT-rich region characteristic of a replication origin. It carries four putative genes that encode a Mob-like, replication initiation (RepAB-like) and one hypothetical protein, this last one being 91% identical to a protein of unknown function, Cjp32, from the C. *jejuni* virulence plasmid, pVir [21].

Perspectives about Campylobacter Genomic Informations

Comprehensive genome analysis of *Campylobacter* has provided essential information concerning the biology of these organisms. We can suppose that the future delivery of at least 13 new genomes will help to continue extracting important information such as presence of non coding regulatory RNAs, as yet not or only poorly described.

Chapter IV

From Environment to the Host: Stress Resistance Mechanisms and Regulation Pathways

3.1. Survival of *Campylobacter jejuni* in Unfavourable Environments: Responses to Starvation and Osmotic Stress

Introduction

The Gram-negative bacterium *Campylobacter jejuni* is a commensal in lot of animals especially in birds [250]. *C. jejuni*, however, is a human gastroenteritis pathogen, and could be considered responsible for as many as 400–500 million cases worldwide each year [117]. Even if intestinal tracts are the natural niche of *Campylobacter jejuni*, this bacterium may be isolated in other hostile environments such as air, water, and soil [51] indicating some survival capacities. One proposed strategy for survival is the controversial viable but non cultivable stage, which would need to to correspond to mechanisms involved in stress responses, especially those generated by hypo-osmotic environment and starvation.

3.1.1. Viable but Not Cultivable Cells of *Campylobacter jejuni*

The concept of viable but not cultivable cells (VBNC) was developed after observations of variations between bacterial counts on classical media and those using microscopic methods. The difficulty is to know exactly in which physiological state the non cultivable bacteria are: lethally injured, in a degenerescent way, or in a strategically survival state. In 1987 Roszak and Colwell [323] proposed the VBNC concept to describe non cultivable bacteria conserving metabolic activities. These VBNC-cells could be resuscitated when placed in a favourable environment such as digestive tract.

The detection of VBNC cells is based on the demonstration of physiological activities such as the ability to replicate DNA, a metabolic activity or cellular integrity compared to multiplication. There are different methods reported for identification of VBNC and the most frequently employed are described below. The cellular elongation assay [196] is based on the use of a media containing low concentrations of nutrients and an inhibitor of cellular division. This leads to distinguishable viable cells, which are able to assimilate nutrients, and subsequently elongate from dead cells, which conserve their initial morphologies. The second technique is based on evidence of an enzymatic activity especially in the electron-transport chain. In 1992, Rodriguez *et al.* [318] proposed a formazan salt (5-cyano-2,3-ditolyl tetrazolium chloride (CTC)), which gives a fluorescent precipitate easily detectable inviable cells. This method, combined with 4-6 diamino 2-phenylindole (DAPI), was employed by Cappelier *et al.* [60] to monitor VBNC cells of *C. jejuni*. The third most used method corresponds to the Live/Dead kit, which employs two nucleic acid stains: viable bacteria with intact membranes fluoresce green, while damaged cells fluoresce red. The use of these methods on a bacterial population show the existence of numerous subpopulations which evolve over time [177].

Entry into the VBNC phase depends on numerous factors. Low availability of nutrients or entry into stationary phase are the conditions where *Campylobacter* species have been shown to become viable but non culturable [22, 43, 169, 319, 378]. Another important factor is the temperature at which starved cells are assayed. Transition to the non cultivable stage occurs more rapidly at high temperatures (from 2 days at 37°C to more than 2 weeks at 4°C) [169, 281, 373, 380]. The exposure to UV has also an influence on the loss of cultivability of strains of *Campylobacter* spp. [281]. In addition, temperature affects the physiological state before the application of starvation. Duffy and Dykes [97] observed a greater decrease in number of cultivable cells in strains previously grown at 42°C as compared with 37°C. The composition of gas mixture, especially a high level of oxygen affects also the cultivability of *C. jejuni* [45].

The concept of VBNC cells includes the controversial ability to resuscitate *in vitro* and *in vivo*. To our knowledge, *in vitro*-resuscitation of *C. jejuni* VBNC has not been described to date. Animal-models used to demonstrate the recovery of VBNC cells show the ability of such cells to colonize [174, 329, 371, 378]. Other researchers have observed that VBNC cells were not always recovered, so they have suggested that such cells of *C. jejuni* are in a degenerative form unable to be resuscitated [246]. These divergent observations could be due to either the way used to obtain VBNC cells, the age of these cells or the strain diversity in *C. jejuni* as reported by Talibart *et al.* [371].

Some physiological modifications are observed in the VBNC cells of *C. jejuni*. The morphological changes correspond to a subsequent elongation followed by the appearance of coccoid forms which are now considered as degenerative forms [189, 379]. Moreover, the maintenance of long-term viability in starved cells is shown to be associated with vibrioid cells [60, 109]. Cytosol condensation is also observed in the VBNC cells. Global molecular changes are identified in the survival mechanism of *C. jejuni* and are related to protein, lipid and polysaccharide-oligo-saccharide compositions [254]. Although it has not been described in *C. jejuni*, oxidation of proteins was detected in VBNC cells of *E. coli* underlying this phenomenon as a significant physiological trait of such cells [89].

Even if VBNC cells could be considered as injured cells, *C. jejuni* seems able to potentially overcome unfavourable environments. In this case, survival mechanisms would correspond to the response of this bacterium to cold temperature (see §3.3), starvation, osmotic changes, and also oxidative stress (see §3.2).

3.1.2. Osmoadaptation of *Campylobacter jejuni*

The term osmoadaptation represents both physiological and genetic adaptations to low and high water environments [122].

The primary bacterial response to osmotic shock is to increase levels of K^+ and its counter-ion contributor, which is glutamate in *E. coli* [244]. This accumulation of K^+ is mediated by four low- and one high- affinity K^+ transport systems (reviewed in [347]). *C. jejuni* possesses at least one transporter and a cluster of genes comprising, some but not all, genes encoding the high-affinity system [292]. The secondary response corresponds to the accumulation of neutral osmoprotectants. Three compounds namely glycine betaine, carnitine and proline are the principal compatible solutes (reviewed in [347]). The preferred osmoprotectant for the majority of prokaryotes is glycine betaine, which accumulates either by neosynthesis or by uptake (BetA-BetB and ProP/ProU systems in *E. coli*). Outer membrane porins also play a role because they facilitate the non-specific diffusion of small hydrophilic molecules (reviewed in [347]). Non-accumulating disaccharides were also identified by Gouffi and Blanco [129] as a new class of sinorhizobial osmoprotectants. Concerning *C. jejuni*, we have been unable to find any study related to hyper-osmotic adaptation. This could be due to the fact that *C. jejuni* is sensitive to salted media and does not grow at NaCl levels of 1.5% [187]. Moreover, osmoprotectant systems homologous to BetAB, GbsAB, OtsAB, and ProP are not found in this micro-organism [294].

Hypo-osmotic shock leads to a massive influx of water in the cell. In order to avoid cell lysis, bacteria have evolved a number of mechanisms for solute and water efflux. Mechanosensitive or stretch-activated channels contribute to the release of cytoplasmic solutes to achieve a rapid reduction of turgor pressure. *E. coli* possesses between three and five stretch-activated channels, the best characterised of which are MscL and MscS (reviewed in [347]). In *Campylobacter jejuni*, there is a protein (Cj0238) which shows similarity to a protein of the epsilon proteobacterium *Helicobacter pylori*, which belongs to the mcsS family [237]. Nevertheless, there is no experimental evidence about the response of *C. jejuni* to low osmolarity. Bacteria possess aquaporin (AqpZ in *E. coli*); a specific channel that is involved in water flux [58]. No obvious homologue for this class of protein has been found in *C. jejuni*.

3.1.3. *Campylobacter jejuni* and Starvation

When many bacteria are grown in standard laboratory media, the cells grow exponentially and enter stationary phase, or starvation. The bacteria undergo structural and physiological changes, which correspond to the establishment of a global stress response that allows resistance to numerous stresses (oxidative, osmotic, acid). In *E. coli*, there is a stationary-phase sigma factor RpoS that controls about fifty genes, which is absent in the genomes of *Campylobacter* species [113, 294].

Contrary to other bacteria, the resistance of *Campylobacter* species to different stresses is not enhanced during the stationary phase. Cells taken from the stationary phase were found to be more sensitive to mild heat stress, aeration, and acid than cells of the exponential phase [189, 264]. However, Cappelier *et al.* [61] reported an increase in heat shock resistance in *C. jejuni* starved cells which did not occur in presence of a protein synthesis inhibitor.

Different physiological modifications were observed when cells of *C. jejuni* were submitted to starvation. Martinez-Rodriguez *et al.* [240] pointed out that cells entered into stationary phase display a change in the fatty-acids composition of their membranes. The ability of *C. jejuni* to modify its membrane fatty acid composition on entry into stationary phase is consistent with the fact that this organism can modulate its membrane composition subsequent to changes in temperature or growth rate [147, 160, 206]. However, variations in the acid or heat tolerances of cells entered in stationary phase were observed when the stresses were applied in cell-free spent medium suggesting a protective effect of an extracellular protective compound [264].

The emergence of variants displaying enhanced survival in stationary phase has been demonstrated in *C. jejuni* strains. These variant cells also show an increased resistance to aeration, heat and hydrogen peroxide [239]. In a previous study, Kelly *et al.* [189] reported inconstant numbers of viable cells during the stationary phase of *C. jejuni*. This emergence of new kinds of cells could indicate a survival strategy for *C. jejuni* when it encounters variable environments; similarly to the GASP (growth advantage in stationary phase) mutants described in *E. coli* [413]. In *E. coli*, this GASP phenotype is related to mutations in the *rpoS* or *lrp* gene resulting in attenuated RpoS or inactive LRP, and this increased fitness is dependent on the pH and nutrient environment [107, 417]. In *C. jejuni*, Martinez-Rodriguez *et al.* [239] were unable to clearly demonstrate the conventional GASP phenotype as described in *E. coli*. Nevertheless, the phenotypic changes observed in *C. jejuni* appeared to be stable because they were maintained in subculture suggesting the emergence of a new strain with advantageous properties in terms of survival in starvation.

In order to understand the specific requirements of *C. jejuni*, it is helpful to consider the metabolism and the respiratory chain of this bacterium. The metabolic capabilities of *C. jejuni* are not well known. It is assumed that carbohydrates in general are not utilized. Some variable patterns in substrate utilisation have been observed in different strains [255]. In this study, all the tested strains of *C. jejuni* were unable to metabolize glucose and oxidized formate, L-lactate, cysteine, serine and glutamine. Variations of oxidation concerned 2-oxoglutarate, succinate, fumarate and aspartic acid. However, comparative analysis of the genomes of *C. jejuni* revealed that this bacterium have a complete oxidative tricarboxylic acid cycle [113, 190] that generates biosynthetic compounds and intermediates that feed into electron transport. Except the phosphofructokinase, all enzymes involved in glycolysis are present, and gluconeogenesis seems to be possible [190, 294]. Pathways for the metabolism and biosynthesis of a number of amino acids are present. *C. jejuni* is a microaerophilic bacteria with a respiratory metabolism based on the use of oxygen as the terminal electron acceptor. The sequence of the genome reveals components of aerobic respiratory chain, namely dehydrogenases, cytochrome bc1 complex and two terminal oxidases [168, 190]. Nevertheless, anaerobic respiration seems possible with other alternative electron acceptors (fumarate, nitrate, hydrogen, formate, and others organics acids) [190]. The respiratory chain in *C. jejuni* is highly branched and complex and it is clear that this bacterium retains an enzymatic equipment allowing flexibility with respect to the variety of electron donors and acceptors.

In numerous bacterial species, the stringent response has been shown to occur in reaction to amino-acid starvation or carbon starvation and to affect various functions to coordinate cellular process. Most bacteria require the stringent response for stationary phase survival [64] or resistance to specific stress [305]. Gaynor *et al.* [124] clearly demonstrated the existence of a stringent response in *C. jejuni* that is required for several specific stress including stationary phase survival, growth and survival under low carbon dioxide/high oxygen levels, and antibiotic resistance-related phenotypes.

In *E. Coli* and other enterobacteria, the catabolic repression via the camp-CRP system allows alternative use of carbon sources [42]. In *C. jejuni*, the existence of a catabolic repression is compromised by the fact that the only homologue of the CRP/FNR family (*cj0466*) seems only to be involved in the resistance to the nitric oxide stress [102].

In order to face nutriment starvation, bacteria accumulate reserves such as glycogen or inorganic polyphosphates with a phosphoanhydric link rich in energy [200]. The nature of accumulated reserves in *C. jejuni* is still unknown, however granules of inorganic polyphosphate were observed in the cytosol of this bacterium [292]. They would potentially serve as an energy source as it has been shown in *H. pylori* [278].

Phosphorus is an essential compound and plays a central role in synthesis of biomolecules and in catabolic processes. In *E. coli*, the expression of proteins involved in assimilation of inorganic phosphate or degradation of either organophosphates or phosphonates is regulated by a two component system (TCR) named Pho BR. In *C. jejuni*, a TCR PhosS/PhosR, not similar to the *E. coli* system, was recently described [406] to be involved in responses to Pi limitation and to activate the pstSCAB genes and eight other genes including a phosphatase gene (*cj0145*) and genes with functions to be determined. These authors propose that the PhosS/PhosR system could be needed to survive in less favoured *Campylobacter* habitats because this system is not involved in colonisation in the chicken gut. The two-component regulatory systems allow a physiological response of bacteria to changing environmental conditions (for further information, see §3.5.3).

As it was mentioned above, in many bacteria, the sigma factor RpoS regulates stationary- phase genes and is considered as a global stress response. There is not any homologue in *C. jejuni*. However, genes involved in the growth stage are regulated during starvation [254]. A possible survival mechanism may be to down regulate as many genes as possible to save energy and to up regulate genes involved in energy metabolism and modification of the cell wall components. The Csr (Carbon storage regulator) could be a global regulatory system that controls the expression of these genes at the post-translational level [320]. In *H. pylori*, CsrA has a broad role in regulating its physiology in response to environmental stimuli [25]. *C. jejuni* possesses a homologue of CsrA, which could be a key regulator in starvation to mediate the reorientation of the metabolism and to cope with other regulators (Fur and HspR) as it was shown in *H. pylori*.

Conclusion

Campylobacter jejuni is considered as a fragile and sensitive bacterium. This discords with the ability of *C. jejuni* to survive to unfavourable environments such as water and also in the food chain. *C. jejuni* shows deficiency in some adaptive mechanisms such as those controlled by RpoS, and the osmoadaptation insufficiently studied. This bacterium possesses (i) metabolic potentialities and a lissom respiratory system, not completely elucidated, that would be functions of ability to occupy different niches, and (ii) a minimal regulatory system for functions involved in the adaptation to hostile environments that suggests alternative survival strategies different from the well known mechanisms described in bacterial models.

3.2. Oxidative Stress in a Microaerophilic Pathogen: Comparison with Aerobic/Anaerobic Microorganisms

Oxidative stress is of particular interest in food safety, as pathogens inevitably enter in contact with ambient air during transmission from their niche to their host or during the food process. It constitutes a strategy against the attack of pathogenic bacteria used naturally by macrophages but also by food industry and medicine [385, 415], [283]. Production of ROS is also stimulated by numerous antibiotics [128]. The tolerance of these pathogens to oxygen depends on their specific defence response that could be related to their aerobic, microaerophilic or anaerobic character. Indeed, anaerobic microorganisms are not exposed to ROS produced by aerobic respiration and their oxygen sensitivity is likely to be related to a lack of detoxification mechanisms. However, if some anaerobes are very sensitive to aerobic conditions, some others, like *Bacteroides fragilis*, can survive long periods of aeration [315]. The aim of this work is to review the different defence strategies developed by bacteria against oxidative stress, conferring them their more or less high resistance in ambient air or inside their host, and conditioning their virulence.

3.2.1. Effect of Oxidative Stress on the Cell

3.2.1.1. Reactivity of the Different Oxygen Species

Farr and Kogoma, in 1991, [106] have defined oxidative stress as an excess of prooxidants in the cell. These prooxidants are mainly reactive oxygen species (ROS), such as superoxide anions, (O_2^-), hydrogen peroxide (H_2O_2) or hydroxyl radicals ($OH^\bullet$). They damage proteins, nucleic acids and cell membranes. Superoxide anion (O_2^-) is very selective and has a moderate oxidative strength due to its negative charge, but can diffuse a long distance before it reacts. Spontaneous dismutation of O_2^- forms $H_2O_2 + O_2$. Hydrogen peroxide (H_2O_2) is a weak oxidizing agent, but it rapidly forms hydroxyl radicals (OH°) through the Fenton reaction, in association with transition metals like free iron. Unlike H_2O_2 and O_2^-, OH° are very reactive but are unable to diffuse a long distance through the cell [115]. Iron plays a critical role in oxidative damages, as it contributes to the formation of highly reactive species through the Haber-Weiss or Fenton reactions, giving rise to hydroxyl radicals.

$$H_2O_2 \xrightarrow{Fe^{2+}/Fe^{3+}} OH° + OH^- \qquad \text{Fenton reaction}$$

$$H_2O_2 + O_2^- \xrightarrow{Fe^{2+}/Fe^{3+}} OH° + OH^- + O_2 \qquad \text{Haber-Weiss reaction}$$

Iron-oxygen complexes, named perferryl radicals $[2Fe^{2+}O_2]°$, are formed from superoxide anions and Fe^{3+}. These complexes are unable to oxidize biomolecules, but rapidly form ferryl radicals $[2Fe^{2+}O]°$, considered as major initiators of lipid peroxidation and DNA damage. Ozone, which is a common air pollutant, is also part of the highly reactive oxygen species. It reacts directly with dienes, amines and thiols, or decomposes to $OH°$ and $HOO°$ [106].

3.2.1.2. Damages

Effects on Proteins

Proteins that contain metal ions at their active sites are highly susceptible to hydroxyl or ferryl radicals. This results in the alteration of the protein function, as changes occur in the protein conformation [112]. Hydroxyl radicals attack the protein backbone to form carbon-centered radicals, which rapidly react with O_2, giving rise to alkyl, alkylperoxide and alkoxyl radicals. These radicals are capable of reacting with other amino acids (of the same protein or not) to form new carbon-centered radicals. Two carbon-centered radicals react with each other in the absence of oxygen to form a protein-protein cross-linkage. Alkoxyl radicals are also responsible for protein fragmentation.

Hydroxyl radicals also oxidize amino acid residue side chains and are involved in the formation of carbonyl residues. All amino acid residues are susceptible, but some residues as lysine, proline, arginine or cysteine are particularly susceptible, giving rise to semialdehydes, acids or disulfides. Peroxynitrite, obtained from nitric oxide and $O_2°^-$, is also responsible for amino acids oxidation, particularly methionine and cysteine (containing sulfur), and for irreversible tyrosine nitration in the presence of CO_2 [30]. All these reactions have consequences on transport systems or enzyme activities. It has been demonstrated that the change of a single histidine residue in an asparagine in the catalytic site caused the loss of catalytic activity in *E. coli* glutamine synthetase

[12, 105]. Oxidation of amino acid residues, protein cleavage or reactions with aldehydes produced after lipid peroxidation lead to the formation of carbonyl residues, which are used as markers of protein oxidation by ROS [12, 252].

Some dehydratases, like aconitase, contain [4 Fe-4S] cluster to bind and dehydrate substrates. It has been demonstrated in *E. coli* that superoxide anions ($O_2^{\circ-}$), obtained from the conjugated form of O_2^-, inactivate these enzymes by oxidatively destroying their iron-sulfur clusters. This causes the inability of the organism to catabolise non-fermentable carbon sources and the release of free iron in the cytosol [116, 363].

Effects on Lipids and Membranes

In membranes, hydroxyl radicals initiate the peroxidation of polyunsaturated fatty acids (see figure 1), leading to the formation of radicals. These radicals react with other fatty acids or with membrane proteins, causing chain reactions. Some intermediates and products of the different steps of lipid peroxidation are highly oxidative compounds, like malondialdehyde. This compound reacts with phospholipids, nucleic acids or proteins and modifies their structure, forming inter- and intra- molecular bridges [123].

Initiation

$$LH + OH^\circ \rightarrow L^\circ + H_2O$$

Propagation

$$L^\circ + O_2 \rightarrow LOO^\circ$$

$$LOO^\circ + LH \rightarrow LOOH + L^\circ$$

Hydroperoxide decomposition

$$LOOH \rightarrow LO^\circ \rightarrow Malondialdehyde$$

LH : polyunsaturated fatty acid ; L° : alkyl radical ; LOOH : lipid hydroperoxide ; LO° : alkoxyl radical.

Figure 1. Mechanism of lipid peroxidation.

Membranes are sensitive to oxidation by both reactive oxygen/nitrogen species. Ozone can react with polyunsaturated fatty acids to form cyclic peroxides, H_2O_2 and aldehydes [106]. Studies on model and mitochondrial membranes have shown that oxidative attack of phospholipids led to changes in the phospholipids organisation, and to perturbation of the lipid bilayer, possibly leading to membrane breakdown [247].

Effects on DNA

Through the Fenton reaction and the production of hydroxyl radicals, H_2O_2 and O_2^- are responsible for DNA alteration. By destroying the iron-sulfur clusters of dehydratases, the accumulation of $O_2^{°-}$ is responsible for the release of a high rate of free cytosolic iron. Metal cations adhere to polyanionic structures like DNA and cellular membranes, constituting the first targets of hydroxyl radicals, which can oxidize DNA by attacking both sugar and base moieties [115, 191]. Most of the damages on DNA are caused by singlet oxygen and hydroxyl radicals. Both purine and pyrimidine bases, so as nucleotides, are oxidized. Single and double-stranded breaks can occur [404]. Mutagenesis and carcinogenesis are caused by the attack of hydroxyl radicals on guanine [123].

3.2.2. Oxidative Stress Responses in Aerobes, Anaerobes and Microaerophiles

Due to its high redox potential and ubiquity, oxygen is used as an electron acceptor in many metabolic pathways. As by-products of oxygen reactions are toxic to the cell, microorganisms using oxygen have to own specific detoxification systems to prevent serious damages to occur [52]. Microorganisms can be classified in five major groups as regards their sensitivity level or need for oxygen, described in table 8 [384].

Bacillus subtilis is a strict aerobe needing high oxygen tensions for growth, whereas *Clostridium perfringens* and *Bacteroides fragilis* are aerotolerant or strict anaerobes, growing only at $pO_2<$ 0.5-2%. *Campylobacter jejuni*, like *Helicobacter pylori*, is considered a microaerophilic bacterium. It grows at oxygen tensions 5-10% and requires relatively high carbon dioxide tensions (3-15%). Indeed, microaerophily can be related to capnophily (need for carbon dioxide) [198].

Table 8. Five Major Groups of Microorganisms Classified by Oxygen Dependance/Tolerance

	Strict Aerobes	Microaerophiles	Facultative Anaerobes	Aerotolerant Anaerobes	Strict Anaerobes
Use of O_2	yes	yes	yes	no	no
pO_2 for growth	21% O_2	5-10% O_2, sensitivity to atmospheric oxygen conditions	O_2 tolerant, no need for growth	O_2 tolerant	Grow only at $pO_2 < 0,5-2\%$

Recently, by showing that for growth of *H. pylori*, need for high CO_2 tension was more important than low oxygen tension, Bury-Moné et al. [52] wondered if *H. pylori* could really be classified as a microaerophile. Antioxidant systems of *H. pylori* were reviewed by Wang et al. [397], who said "the oxidative stress response of *H. pylori* is much more vast, adaptable and interconnected than previously appreciated". The comparison of oxidative stress resistance related to detoxification and regulation systems present in a strict aerobe (*B. subtilis*), a facultative anaerobe (*E. coli*), microaerophilic bacteria (*C. jejuni* and *H. pylori*) and anaerobes (*C. perfringens* and *Bacteroides fragilis*) are here reviewed to conclude on the *C. jejuni* legitimacy as an oxidative stress sensitive microorganism.

3.2.2.1. Effect of Atmospheric Oxygen and ROS on Survival

Oxygen Tension

Aerobiosis constitutes the optimal atmospheric condition for growth of strict aerobes. Incubation of *Campylobacter jejuni* under aerobic conditions results in a decrease of 2 Log_{10} of the total population between 6 and 12 h, and then a rapid decrease of 5 more Log_{10} between 12 and 15 h. During the first 6 hours, no loss of viability is observed, and this can be correlated with the expression of a protein whose molecular weight could correspond to superoxide dismutase or alkyl hydroperoxide reductase [410]. Recent studies on chicken breast fillets showed that a nitrogen/carbon dioxide mixture or an oxygen-enriched atmosphere led to a more significant decrease in *C. jejuni* population than vacuum or ambient air [45, 224]. It has been shown that on solid media, *H. pylori* is able to grow in aerobic conditions (but at lower rates than in optimal conditions). No differences in protein profiles were observed between samples from aerobic and microaerobic cultures. When CO_2 tension increases, *H. pylori* is no longer sensitive to oxygen.

Indeed, many laboratories use atmospheres containing 19-20% O_2 and 5-10% CO_2 for growth of *H. pylori* [52]. *C. perfringens* liquid cultures are unable to grow in aerobic conditions and show a rapid decrease in survival (2 to 3 Log_{10} decrease within the first 2 hours) [47, 282]. In *B. fragilis* cultures, aerobic conditions do not lead to a significant decrease in population within the first 48 hours. It leads to a 6 Log_{10} population reduction after 70 hours, whereas less than a 1 Log_{10} reduction is observed in anaerobic cultures [315].

Superoxide Stress

Different chemicals can be used as superoxide anions generators in the cell to assess their superoxide stress resistance, like plumbagin, menadione, cumene hydroperoxide or paraquat [106]. Paraquat, also named methyl viologen, is the most used superoxide generator, catalysing electron transfer from redox enzymes to oxygen [363]. Data are available on paraquat resistance of the microorganisms considered here, but a comparison is hardly possible, as different techniques are employed (liquid cultures or disk diffusion assays on agar plates) [106, 172, 372, 394]. Concerning *C. jejuni*, paraquat has been used to characterize superoxide stress sensitive mutants but the low concentrations applied allowed growth of the wild strain [394]. It would be interesting to have more comparable data on *C. jejuni* superoxide stress resistance.

Hydrogen Peroxide

H_2O_2 is commonly used as a chemical agent for studies on oxidative stress resistance. It has been described that inside the host, H_2O_2 concentration in phagocytes can reach 100 µM [289]. In mid-log phase *B. subtilis* cultures, the effect of a 50 µM treatment on the culture survival is negligible [266]. Addition of 116 µM H_2O_2 or 100 µM paraquat (superoxide stress) to a mid-log phase culture leads to a decrease in growth rate but not in population [372]. It was also shown that 15 min exposure to 1 mM H_2O_2 had no effect on total population [38]. After incubating *C. jejuni* cultures with 1 or 0.5 mM H_2O_2 during 15 min, a 4 Log_{10} decrease in the total population has been observed, showing that this bacterium is highly susceptible to peroxide stress. After 4 hours at 1 mM, no bacteria was detected, whereas the initial level of population was recovered after 2-4 h at 0.5 mM. It was suggested that the bacteria rapidly recovered a growth-competent state from a non-culturable state [410]. Unlike *C. jejuni*, *H. pylori* appears quite resistant to hydrogen peroxide. No decline in survival was observed for *H. pylori* cultures exposed to 98 mM hydrogen peroxide in different iron availability conditions. However, unlike the results presented for the other bacteria, these observations were obtained from stationary-phase cultures [141]. Indeed, despite the absence of a RpoS general regulator in *C. jejuni* and *H. pylori*, the shift from exponential to stationary phase could lead to specific gene regulations, namely through the stringent response [262](see below in Regulation Pathways). A 15 min treatment with 50 µM H_2O_2 has no effect on *B. fragilis* population and a 1 Log_{10} population reduction can be observed after 15 min exposure to 1 mM H_2O_2 [315]. Mid-log phase *C. perfringens* cultures are not significantly inhibited by 50 µM H_2O_2, whereas a 1 Log_{10} and a 4 Log_{10} decrease in population is observed when exposed to 100 µM and 150 µM respectively [47].

Whereas *H. pylori* is resistant to both oxygen and hydrogen peroxide, *C. jejuni* is clearly more sensitive to oxidative stress than aerobic and even than some anaerobic bacteria.

Spores and Viable but Non Culturable Forms

In Bacilli and Clostridia, stress leads to formation of highly resistant dormant cells, called spores. These quiescent spores are surrounded by a specific protein structure, called coat, which allows survival to very severe stresses. This coat itself is surrounded by additional structures, like exosporia (made of proteins, glycoproteins and lipids) or different appendages of unknown functions [96].

As it has been described above (see §3.1), in unfavourable conditions, *C. jejuni*, like many Gram negative bacteria, is able to adopt a coccoid form which is called viable but non culturable (VBNC). It has been demonstrated that a culture in presence of hydrogen peroxide contained coccoid forms and that the number of these forms was reduced when superoxide dismutase or a superoxide anion scavenging enzyme was added to the culture [257]. In 1998, Harvey and Leach [144] have demonstrated that in continuous cultures of *C. jejuni*, the transformation of coccoid forms was only observed with high oxygen tension when it is combined with reduced carbon concentrations. However, the medium used contained protective agents against oxygen toxicity. Unlike what has been described for Bacilli and Clostridia spores, no specific external structures are observed on VBNC forms, which are often considered as degenerated forms [291]. VBNC forms have also been described for *H. pylori* cultures in aerobic (21% O_2) and anaerobic (<1% O_2) conditions, and for *E. coli* during nutrient starvation. In these microorganisms, VBNC forms showed high protein oxidative damage, decreased levels of catalase and SOD activities (as a consequence), as well as high DNA damage level and mutagenicity, suggesting that they may be consequences of deterioration rather than an adaptative response [89, 288].

3.2.2.2. Resistance Mechanisms

The major proteins involved in oxidative stress defence and their known regulation systems are summarized in table 9. Complete genome sequences are available for all microorganisms considered here. For some genes, indication of their absence or presence was confirmed after interrogating the KEGG [180].

Detoxification

Superoxide Stress

Superoxide dismutase (SOD) is an enzyme, co-factored by different metallic ions, converting superoxide anions into hydrogen peroxide and dioxygen. *B. subtilis* codes for a single manganese superoxide dismutase [65], whereas *E. coli* codes for 3 SODs (MnSOD, FeSOD, Cu/ZnSOD) [363, 372]. *C. jejuni*, like *H. pylori*, codes for a single superoxide dismutase, SodB, cofactored by iron [302, 389]. SOD seems to be involved in survival of *C. jejuni* in epithelial cells [301]. The principal resistance mechanism used by epithelial cells against bacterial attacks consists in the action of postinflammatory cytokins, activating the nitric synthase isozyme and leading to the production of nitric oxides. By eliminating superoxides, SOD prevents their reaction with nitric oxides [385]. In *H. pylori*, it has been demonstrated that the FeSOD was partially located at the surface of the bacteria, and also on the flagella, but such locations for *C. jejuni* FeSOD have not been described [302]. Interestingly, in *B. subtilis*, no change in SodA expression was observed after exposure to paraquat (a superoxide-forming agent) [372]. In 1987, Scott *et al.* had already shown in *E. coli* that an overproduction of SOD did not result in increased resistance to superoxide stress, but even resulted in increased susceptibility, due to H_2O_2 accumulation [340]. *C. perfringens*, like *B. fragilis*, possesses a single Mn-SOD. Two rubredoxins were suspected to be part of alternative superoxide reductase systems, first described for *Desulfovibrio vulgaris*, but no activity of this system has been observed [172, 225].

Table 9. Proteins involved in oxidative stress defence and their known regulation systems

Function	B. subtilis			E. coli			C. jejuni			H. pylori			B. fragilis			C. perfringens		
		gene	regulon		gene	regulon		gene	regulon		gene	regulon		gene	regulon		gene	regulon
Alkyl Hydroperoxide reductase (small subunit)	+	ahpC	PerR	+	ahpC	OxyR	+	ahpC	PerR	+	ahpC	CsrA	+	ahpC	OxyR	+	ahpC	
Alkyl Hydroperoxide reductase (large subunit)	+	ahpF	PerR	+	ahpF	OxyR							+	ahpF	OxyR	-		
Catalase	+	katA	PerR, σE	+	katG	OxyR, σS	+	katA	PerR	+	katA	Fur	+	katB	OxyR	-		
	+	katE	σB	+	katE	σS												
KatA-associated protein										+	kapA							
Cytochrome c peroxidase							+	ccp	RacS/RacR, PerR				+	ccp	OxyR			
Metalloregulation DNA-binding stress protein	+	mrgA	PerR	+	dps	OxyR, σS	+	dps	PerR, Fur				+	dps	OxyR	-		
Ferric Uptake regulator	+	fur		+	fur	SoxRS, OxyR	+	fur	PerR	+	fur	CsrA				+	furR	
PerR	+	perR					+	perR	PerR	-								
OxyR	-			+	oxyR	OxyR	-			-								
Superoxide radical response R protein	-			+	soxR					-								

Function	B. subtilis		E. coli		C. jejuni		H.pylori		B. fragilis		C. perfringens	
	gene	regulon	gene	regulon	gene	regulon	gene	regulon	gene	regulon	gene	regulon
Superoxide radical response S protein	-		+	soxS	-		-					
LexA	+	lexA	+	lexA	-		-		-		+	lexA
Manganese superoxide dismutase	+	sodA	+	sodA	Spx, σB	SoxRS, Fur					+	sodA
Iron superoxide dismutase	-		+	sodB	small RNA RyhB	+	sodB	PerR	+	sodB	Fur	
Copper-Zinc superoxide dismutase	-		+	sodC	σS							
Multifunctional SOS repair regulator	+	recA	RecA/LexA	+	recA	RecA/LexA					+	rexA
Excinuclease ABC (subunit B)	+	uvrB	RecA/LexA	+	uvrB							+	uvrB
Methionine sulfoxide reductase	+	msrA		+	msrA		+	msrA					
	+	msrB	small RNA RyhB	+	msrB	small RNA RyhB	+	msrB					
Thiol peroxidase	+	tpx	Spx	+	tpx		+	tpx		+	tagD	+	tpx	-	
Thioredoxin	+	trxA	Spx, σB	+	trxC	oxyR	+	trxA		+	trxA		+	trxl	+	trxl
thioredoxin reductase	+	yegT	Fur, Spx	+	trxB		+	trxB	PerR	+	trxB		+	trxR	+	trxR
References	[372]		[363] [416]		[389]		[397]		[156]		[172]	

Peroxide Stress

Catalase activity represents the main peroxide stress defence. The genome of *Bacillus subtilis* contains genes coding for 2 different catalases [222]. Engelmann, in 1996 has shown that KatA is specifically induced in oxidative stress conditions, whereas KatE is a general stress response protein (sigmaB dependant) [103]. *E. coli* also expresses two catalases (HPI catalase encoded by *katG* and HPII encoded by *katE*) and only HPI is specifically induced in presence of H_2O_2 [363]. *C. jejuni* and *H. pylori* code for a single heme-cofactored catalase, KatA [149, 389]. In *H. pylori*, this catalase is present in both cytoplasm and periplasm [142]. Day *et al.* (2000) have demonstrated that in *C. jejuni*, catalase was not involved in cell survival but played a role in intramacrophage survival, as *katA* mutants survival is unaffected in epithelial cells but limited in macrophages [81]. In *H. pylori* catalase deficient mutants, survival in presence of exogenous ROS produced by professional phagocytes and macrophages is also reduced [27, 311]. However, *H. pylori* catalase seems to have unique features. Downstream of the *katA* gene is a gene coding for KapA (KatA-associated protein) involved in periplasmic hydrogen peroxide resistance [141]. No homologue has been found in any other related or unrelated species. The role of this KapA protein seems to be highly significant. Indeed, whereas a wild strain shows no decrease in survival at 100 mM H_2O_2, a *kapA*-mutant shows a very rapid decline [141]. It has also been shown that *H. pylori* catalase, unlike others, was sensitive to organic hydroperoxides, was unable to bind NADPH and used formic acid instead [223, 397]. No catalase has been found in *C. perfringens* [47] and *B. fragilis* expresses one catalase [315].

In *B. subtilis* and *E. coli*, the alkyl hydroperoxide reductase, converting hydroperoxides into alcohols, is composed of a catalytic (AhpC) and a recycling (AhpF) subunit. Homologues of AhpC are present in *C. jejuni* and *H. pylori*, but no homologue of the AhpF subunit could be found. It has been suggested the role of AhpF could be played by thioredoxin reductases (TrxA and TrxB homologues) [389]. FdxA, located downstream of AhpC in *C. jejuni* genome, has also been proposed to play this role [287].

Thiol peroxidases (Tpx and Bcp in *C. jejuni*) are also involved, protecting proteins from oxidation by glutamine synthetase [389]. They are absent in the aerobe *C. perfringens*.

Iron Homeostasis

As it has been described above, iron, which is an essential element for living organisms, is also responsible for ROS formation through the Fenton and Haber-Weiss reaction. Oxidation of [Fe-S] cluster-containing proteins leads to an increase of intracellular free iron. As a consequence, it is not surprising that oxidative stress and iron uptake regulations overlap and that transcription of genes encoding catalase and AhpC are affected by iron concentration [389]. A ferredoxin (FdxA) was also shown to be involved in *C. jejuni* aerotolerance [388] and a ferritin-deficient mutant is more sensitive to H_2O_2 and paraquat than the parent strain [394].

DNA Protection and Repair

As described above, oxidative stress leads to DNA damage. Specific systems are induced in oxidative stress conditions to protect and repair the genetic information. Dps (DNA-binding protein from starved cells) has been shown in *E. coli* to sequester DNA to isolate it from different damaging conditions (UV light, acid stress, oxidative stress) [73]. No homologue of Dps has been identified in *C. perfringens*, whereas all other bacteria considered here possess one. They all possess a set of DNA reparation systems (comprising RecA, MutS, UvrA,B,C). In *E. coli* as well as in *B. subtilis*, the importance of RecA activity has been demonstrated after H_2O_2 challenge [38, 62]. However, in *C. jejuni*, many other DNA direct repair, glycosylation, mismatch repair functions and some SOS response genes present in *E. coli* are lacking [294].

Reduction or Elimination of Oxidized Proteins

As described above, methionine, like cystein, is a sulphur-containing amino-acid particularly sensitive to oxidative stress. Methionine Sulfoxide Reductases (Msr) are present in all bacteria considered here. Along with thioredoxin and thioredoxin reductase, they allow reduction of oxidized sulfurs [7]. In *H. pylori*, the Trx1 thioredoxin was also shown to play a role in protection of arginase (inhibiting production of nitric oxide by host cells) against oxidative stress [397]. Oxidoreductases play an important role in *C. jejuni* resistance to oxygen, as their expression is particularly increased under oxidative stress conditions in aerotolerant strains [211]. In *E. coli*, the heat shock response overlaps with the oxidative stress response [416]. It has been demonstrated in *C. jejuni* and *E. coli* that the HtrA protease is also involved in oxidized proteins degradation [48, 345].

3.2.2.3. Regulation Pathways

A general stress response can be observed in most bacteria on entry into stationary phase or after exposure to stress conditions, resulting in an increased resistance to heat, acid or oxidative stress. In *E. coli* and *B. subtilis*, the *rpoS* gene codes for the σ^B sigma factor responsible for this general response which regulates the expression of more than 50 genes [240, 372]. In *B. subtilis*, Thackray *et al.*, 2003, have shown that SigmaM, an extracytoplasmic function sigma factor, was activated after exposure to superoxide stress [377]. This sigma factor protects membrane integrity and is induced in different kind of stresses. Such responses are absent in *C. jejuni* and *H. pylori*, which lack σ^S and other sigma factors usually involved [189, 294, 397]. The only observation made on *C. jejuni* which could correspond to a survival strategy on stationary phase is a change in the membrane fatty acid composition, resulting in high pressure resistance [240].

The stringent response has been well described in *E. coli* as a key regulatory pathway to cope with starvation and other environmental stresses. In *C. jejuni* and *H. pylori*, it has been shown that the stringent response, involved in different stress resistance mechanisms such as adaptation to nutritional deprivation or antibiotic resistance and regulated by SpoT, was involved in long term adaptation to growth in aerobic conditions, as a *spoT* mutant has no particular sensitivity to hydrogen peroxide but is defective for survival under high oxygen concentrations [124, 397]. The CsrA protein (carbon storage regulator) is also involved in survival under oxidative stress in *H. pylori*, in which it regulates other regulators like Fur and the heat shock gene regulator HspR [25]. A gene coding for CsrA is present in *C. jejuni* but the role of this protein in oxidative stress resistance has not been determined yet.

In *B. subtilis* and *E. coli*, the SOS response involved in case of DNA damage is mediated by LexA, which is absent in *C. jejuni* [188, 294].

In *E. coli*, specific responses to peroxide and superoxide stress are mediated by OxyR and SoxRS, respectively. OxyR is a positive regulator activated by oxidation controlling AhpCF, catalase and DPS as well as other detoxifying proteins. SoxRS is a system of two regulatory proteins controlling a set of protein amongst which SODA [106]. An OxyR, but no SoxRS, has also been described in *B. fragilis* [316]. No OxyR or SoxRS have been described in *C. jejuni* or other bacteria considered here.

Fur (Ferric Uptake Regulator) is a metal-cofactored repressor controlling iron homeostasis in the cell. These repressors are composed of a metal-binding C-terminal part and a N-terminal helix-turn-helix motif that binds DNA. Fur senses iron level. In the presence of a sufficient quantity of iron, the Fur homodimer forms Apo-Fur with iron, whose new conformation allows it to bind DNA. No iron-responsive autoregulation of Fur has been observed and a sequence analysis showed no Fur-Box allowing binding of apo-Fur upstream of the *fur* gene. Fur is present in each of the bacteria considered here and is mainly involved in iron homeostasis, regulating iron transport and storage proteins such as in *B. subtilis* [372]. Bsat *et al.*, 1998, have demonstrated the presence of 2 Fur homologues in *B. subtilis*, Fur and PerR [50]. In *E. coli*, Fur expression is known to be regulated by OxyR and SoxRS [363].

PerR senses peroxide stress by metal-catalysed oxidation of histidine residues [208]. In *B. subtilis*, Fuanthong *et al.*, 2002, have shown that not all of the PerR regulon proteins were inducible by H_2O_2. PerR controls MrgA, KatA, Ahpcf, HemAXCDBL and ZosA. The gene encoding PerR is self-repressed and also represses *fur* [120]. Interestingly, no gene coding for a PerR regulator has been found in *H. pylori* [397].

In *C. jejuni*, the superoxide and peroxide stress responses seem to be mainly regulated by the same 2 homologues, Fur and PerR. The number of proteins being part of the *C. jejuni* Fur regulon is lower than that of *B. subtilis* [387]. Fur boxes have been identified upstream of 12 genes coding for iron transport and iron storage/binding proteins. Amongst them is Dps, which seems to be potentially regulated by both PerR and Fur [389].The *C. jejuni katA* gene is regulated by PerR and its expression is induced after exposition to hydrogen peroxide. Like in *B. subtilis*, *ahpC* could be regulated by PerR, as putative Fur and Per boxes have been found upstream this gene. In conditions of iron starvation, iron acquisition is induced, giving rise to reactive oxygen species. The activation of *ahpC* could then permit the detoxification of the cell [24]. There exist two sorts of periplasmic cytochrome c peroxidases (Ccp) in *Campylobacter*, one of these possessing a putative PerR/Fur box. It has been demonstrated that its expression was iron dependent but Fur independent. Computational research of PerR boxes have allowed to predict several other proteins as PerR regulated, but no *in vitro* experiment has demonstrated it yet. Amongst these proteins are TrxB, Dps, SodB, Ccp and PerR itself [389].

In *B. subtilis*, expression of thiol peroxidase, thioredoxin, SOD and other proteins involved in detoxification or iron homeostasis are controlled by a Spx transcription regulator, which is also described for *Enterococcus* and *Listeria* but is absent from other bacteria considered here [372].

In *C. jejuni*, few regulatory genes have been identified. Amongst them, some two-component systems have been characterized and none seems to play a critical role in oxidative stress response regulation. The RacR/RacS system controls cytochrome c peroxidase expression [46]. In *E. coli*, the redox-sensing Aer transducer, along with CheA/CheR, modulates cell's flagellar motor [127]. Proteins involved in such an aerotaxis system have been identified in *C. jejuni* but their functions are not fully described yet [153] (see §4.3).

In *E. coli*, lots of non-coding regulatory small RNAs playing a role in stress regulation have been described. The RyhB small RNA has been shown to interact with Fur to regulate MsrB and SOD expression [241]. To date, no regulation systems mediated by small RNAs have been described in *C. jejuni*.

Conclusion

C. jejuni is more sensitive to oxygen and hydrogen peroxide than *E. coli*, *B. subtilis* and *H. pylori*, which is also a microaerophile but shows a high oxidative stress resistance [52]. It is even more sensitive to oxidative stress than *B. fragilis*, which is described as an oxygen tolerant anaerobe [315].

As described above, *C. jejuni* and *H. pylori* possess a single catalase, whereas 2 are present in both *E. coli* and *B. subtilis*. They also possess a single Fe-SOD, whereas 3 have been identified in *E. coli*. They both lack the alkyl hydroperoxide reductase AhpF recycling subunit, which role is supposed to be played by thioredoxin reductases or a ferredoxin. They also both lack important regulators, like OxyR, SoxRS, Spx, global regulator σ^B or the SOS response regulator LexA. Even though they present the same disadvantages and even though *H. pylori* lacks a PerR regulator present in *C. jejuni*, *H. pylori* appears particularly resistant to oxidative stress. This could partly be related to its catalase unique features and its specific catalase-associated protein (KapA), playing a critical role in peroxide stress resistance [397].

The relatively broad range of *C. jejuni* defence mechanisms, regulation pathways or VBNC cells formation described here partly explain how *C. jejuni* survives in aerobic environments and inside the host and leads to so much campylobacteriosis cases throughout the world. However, lots of putative regulation systems remain to be explored, such as TCS, small RNAs or aerotaxis systems. Barnard *et al.*, 2004, had hypothesized on the importance of posttranscriptional regulations in mediating *H. pylori* oxidative stress response [25].

After considering *C. jejuni* oxidative stress sensitivity, it appears that unlike for *H. pylori*, there is no doubt on *C. jejuni* legitimacy as a true microaerophile.

3.3. Campylobacter Responses to Thermal Stress

Introduction

The *Campylobacter jejuni* growth is considered optimal at 42°C and the lower temperature limit for the growth located between 30-35°C depending on the strain. This limit excludes definitely the capacity of this organism to grow outside of the digestive tract of poultry or other warm-blooded animals. Additionally, it does not normally grow aerobically and is not readily transmitted between humans, yet it is the most frequent food-borne pathogen. To better understand this conundrum, its capacities of survival in thermal stress conditions will be explored in the next paragraphs.

3.3.1. Cold Shock Response

Campylobacters are likely exposed to widely fluctuating temperatures in the farm environment or during food process, and their ability to regulate gene expression in response to temperature is therefore fundamental to their continuing survival. It has been reported that *C. jejuni* survive better at 4°C than at 25°C [36]and It has been previously described that *C. jejuni* is still metabolically active at low temperature. The genome sequencing of NCTC 11168 strain in year 2000 [294]revealed the surprising absence of any genes of cold shock proteins family (CspA), which act as RNA chaperones to protect mRNA from the formation of secondary structures [409]. However, oxygen consumption, catalase activity, ATP generation and protein synthesis were already observed at temperatures as low as 4°C [148]. These results have been recently confirmed and in both case (4 and 25°C), cells survived better under anaerobic conditions than under microaerobic or aerobic conditions [254]. The general trend proposed for the genes expression is that there is a massive down regulation except the genes linked to stress response. A possible survival mechanism may be to down regulate as many genes as possible to save energy and to up regulate genes involved in energy metabolism and modification of the cell wall components. Nethertheless, it has been recently described [285] that, in the same conditions than the previous study, the total amount of carbohydrates increased over time and was not captured by the DNA microarray measurements. The authors concluded that essential mechanisms explaining the survival of its bacterium at non-growth temperatures are not yet fully understood. Moen *et al.* (2005) suggested that the increase in carbohydrates may be due to Osmoregulated Periplasmic Glycans (OPGs), which appear to be important for survival of Gram-negative bacteria under extreme conditions [37]. These results are in agreement with the *C. jejuni* capacity to produce a polysaccharide and a previous study has suggested that this capsule is important for the survival of *C. jejuni* [183].

In the particular case of freezing-thawing many data are available about the survival of *Campylobacter* in media or food (see § 1.1.5.2) but only few studies provide the first steps of understanding of the *Campylobacter* mechanisms of resistance to freeze-thaw stress. Freezing and thawing of living cells result in injuries, and it has been proposed that the injuries are the result of several factors, including ice nucleation and dehydration. In addition oxidative damages have been suggested as a mechanism that contributes to freeze-thaw injuries since it has been predicted that an oxydative burst occurs upon thawing. In comparison with previous studies on *Saccharomyces cerevisae*, Stead and Park (2000) showed the relevant role of SOD (superoxide dismutase) and catalase in resistance of *C.coli* to freeze-thaw stress [356]. These studies provide the first steps in understanding the *C. jejuni* mechanism for cold-shock adaptation but further experiments are needed to better elucidate the general response to cold shock [265].

3.3.2. Heat Shock Response

Campylobacter are considered to be more heat sensitive than most bacteria, including other gram-negative food-borne pathogens, such as *Salmonella* spp. and *Escherichia coli* [164]. In other bacteria species, entry into the stationary phase or exposure to starvation conditions results in increase resistance to heat shock. The central regulator for many of these stationary-phase induced changes in a number of gram-negative bacteria is the σ factor RpoS (see §3.1). The genome of *C. jejuni* lacks the genes encoding the RpoS stationary phase response mechanism [294]. However, considerable variations in heat resistance of *Campylobacter* spp. has been observed with observed D_{55} values from 0.75 min to 3.4 min according to the strains [273, 352]. At this temperature *C. jejuni* demonstrated an approximately exponential decline in CFU with time contrary to *C. coli* which showed first order death kinetics in the temperature range of 48.8-55°C. The amazing stability of DNA and mRNA of heat-treated *Campylobacter* (at temperatures of 95-99°C) excludes the denaturation of these molecules as the direct cause of cell death [366]. But in comparison with previous studies on *B. subtilis* and *E. coli*, Nguyen *et al.* (2006) proposed recently that *Campylobacter* cells death is coincident with heat denaturation of sensitive parts of ribosome and unfolding of alpha and beta subunits of RNA polymerase [273].

In general, exposure of bacteria to stressfull conditions leads to induction of heat-shock proteins separated in two categories, the chaperones and the ATP dependent proteases. These proteins act by repairing and preventing damages caused by accumulation of unfolded proteins. Several of the heat shock proteins also play a crucial role under normal physiological conditions by assisting in the proper folding of newly synthesized proteins. The search for chaperone homologues and heat shock proteins in the *C. jejuni* genome reveals up to 17 proteins, several of which have already been characterized, including GroEL, GroES, DnaJ, DnaK, GrpE, HrcA and Lon [290]. The thermal stress response (from 37 to 46°C) in *C. jejuni* has been characterized, showing the preferential synthesis of 24 proteins immediately following heat shock. The HSP, DnaJ for instance, was considered to play a role *in vivo*, as *C. jejuni* DnaJ mutant was unable to colonize chickens [197]. In addition the heat shock proteins GroEL and GroES are immunogenic in experimentally infected rabbits [408]. These suggest that the heat shock response plays an important role in both thermo-tolerance and also in virulence. More recently, a global gene expression analysis of growth temperature variation (from 37°C to 42°C) showed the different expression of 336 genes during the first 10 min after the shock, whereas less than 50 of these genes remained differently expressed at 50 min [361]. This gene expression pattern suggests that *C. jejuni* is able to adapt to a new steady state at 42°C over time with very few genes differently expressed. Many genes whose expression was altered by temperature encode for proteins of unknown function, thus displaying the limitations in understanding *C. jejuni* physiology. For genes of known function, those encoding proteins involved in energy metabolism, cell wall and envelope constituents and transport are among the most up-regulated genes which suggests a differential surface structure pattern between 42 and 37°C. Genes encoding proteins involved in synthesis and modification of macromolecules are among the most downregulated genes. In addition, the repression of ribosomal genes suggests a brief growth arrest that allows the cell to save and reshuffle energy for repairing damages caused by temperature upshift [361]. The global molecular mechanism of heat shock regulation in *C. jejuni* is still poorly understood. In many other Gram-negative bacteria as *E. coli*, the response to heat stress is positively regulated by an alternative σ^{32} factor, but *C. jejuni* does not possess an homologue of σ^{32} suggesting that its heat shock regulation mechanism is different from that seen in *E. coli*. On the other hand, an alternative complex named HrcA/CIRCE has been identified in more than 40 eubacteria, including proteobacteria [268] as a transcriptional repressor which requires the GroE chaperonin system [314]. Following exposure to stress, GroE levels decreased due to its association to misfolded proteins resulting in decreased binding of HrcA to DNA and activation of heat-shock gene expression. A similar operon, encoding homologues of HrcA (Cj0757), GrpE (Cj0758) and DnaK (Cj0759) is present in the genome of *C. jejuni*.

In contrast with the mechanism described in *B. subtilis*, the heat shock protein DnaJ is absent from this operon but appears elsewhere on the *C. jejuni* chromosome (Cj 1260c) suggesting a alternative regulation system [290]. An other repressor/operator system named HspR/HAIR is less widely utilized in the bacterial kingdom, but has been described in actinomycetes and in *Helicobacter pylori*, an organism closely related to *Campylobacter* [381]. Similarly to HrcA mechanism, environmental stress releases HspR from its DNA-binding element, resulting in expression of the target genes. The analysis of *C. jejuni* genome sequence showed the presence of an homologue of HspR (Cj1230). Andersen *et al.* (2005) have identified 30 members of this regulon by comparison of the proteome and transcriptome of a HspR mutant with a wild type strain. In the absence of HspR, transcripts levels of all genes in the previous hrcA-dnaK-grpE operon were increased indicating a complex interrelationship between HrcA and HspR [13]. These results are in agreement with those described in *H.pylori* where it has been shown that both DnaK and GroEL were co-regulated by HspR and HrcA [354]. Both mechanisms are designed to permit feedback controls at the level of gene expression. *Campylobacter* as many bacteria have established sophisticated regulatory networks, often combining positive and negative mechanisms, in order to allow fine-tuned heat shock gene expression in an environmentally responsive way.

3.4. Responses of *Campylobacter* to Low pH Environments

The human stomach forms a natural barrier for foodborne pathogens. In bacteria like *Salmonella* and *E. coli*, acid resistance mechanisms have evolved which enable them to survive for a prolonged period of time in the human stomach. The induction of these responses, and consequently level of stomach survival, depends on growth phase, and pre-exposure conditions. Besides, stomach survival is affected by the availability of amino acids, by food source [403], and by the rate at which gastric juice is produced [83].

The sensitivity of *Campylobacter jejuni* to acids or acidic environments has not been studied extensively. Like in *Salmonella* and *E. coli*, stress tolerance is affected by medium, but also by growth type (planktonic vs. biofilm growth; [99]). Cell counts of *C. jejuni* rapidly decrease at pH 5 [74]. *C. jejuni* appeared to be highly sensitive to volatile fatty acids [69, 70], and HCl, although to a lesser extent [80]. Yet, it was suggested that *C. jejuni* can induce an adaptive tolerance response to acid conditions [263]. However, this response only results in prolonged survival at pH 4.5. Therefore, the significance of this response remains to be determined, as the pH of the human stomach after consumption of a meal is on average 2.5 [126].

Chapter V

Other Strategies Developed by *Campylobacter* to Adapt to the Environment

4.1. Alteration Of Membrane Lipids

Introduction

The cell membrane constitutes the main barrier to water and solute exchange between the cytoplasm and the external environment. Its flexibility and adaptation capability largely determines the survival ability of the cell [332]. Membranes play an important role in cell physiology as they enable energy transduction through the proton motive force generated by the pH gradient and the transmembrane potential. The cell membrane regulates solutes and ions fluxes to maintain a constant intracellular environment termed as cell homeostasis. To maintain their membrane in the proper lipid bilayer phase (lamellar state) for normal function, bacteria have to adjust their membrane lipid composition in such a way that the membrane fluidity remains constant in response to environmental conditions. Bacterial cytoplasmic membranes can compensate for altered growth conditions by a process known as homeoviscous adaptation which changes the membrane so it can remain in the fluid phase even as the environment changes [343].

4.1.1. Bacterial Membranes

A) General Aspects

Gram-negative bacteria are characteristically bounded by two membranes, the cytoplasmic or inner membrane, which is a phospholipid bilayer, and the outer membrane, which holds phospholipids and lipopolysaccharides (LPS) in its inner and outer leaflet respectively. Both contain numerous proteins that have diverse functions. These membranes, together with the enclosed peptidoglycane-containing periplasm comprise the bacterial cell envelope. The Gram-negative inner membrane carries out a variety of functions typically assigned to both the plasma membrane and specific organelles in higher organisms. These include protein export, solute import, cell signalling, biosynthesis, electron transport, and maintenance of a proton motive force and ATP synthesis.

The outer membrane, consisting of an inner face of phospholipids and an outer face of lipopolysaccharide (LPS), plays an important role in nutrient uptake, but in addition confers resistance to a variety of detergents and antibiotics [93].

B) Bacterial Membrane Lipids

Phospholipid Bilayers

The lipid bilayer forms the framework of the cytoplasmic and the outer membranes. The primary lipid components of this bilayer are the polar glycerophospholipids [313]. Glycerophospholipids are amphipathic molecules constituted by a glycerol molecule esterified by two molecules of fatty acids (lipophilic regions) and one phosphate group, itself ester-bonded to an alcohol group such as serine, ethanolamine, glycerol, choline or inositol (polar head group). Phosphatidylethanolamine and phosphatidylcholine possess an overall neutral charge, while phosphatidylserine and phosphatidylglycerol and cardiolipin (*e.g.* biphosphatidyl glycerol) have an overall negative charge at pH 7.0. Phosphatidylglycerol makes up the greatest percentage of glycerophospholipids in bacterial membranes, whereas phosphatidylcholine and phosphatidylilinositol are rare in prokaryotic membranes [88].

The neutral lipids, hopanoids and carotenoids, modulate membrane fluidity, taking on the same role as sterols (absent in Prokaryotes) in the eukaryotic membrane [325].

The most common membrane fatty acids are 14 to 20 carbons long [328] and even numbered as they are created by multiple additions of two carbons to the carboxyl terminus by an elongase or fatty acid synthetase [324]. However uneven numbered acyl chains exist [327]. Typically, glycerophospholipids have one saturated and one unsaturated fatty acid (UFA). Unsaturated chains may contain up to six *cis*-double bonds; however, polyunsaturation is rare in bacterial membranes [326], occurring mostly in marine psychrophiles and cyanobacteria [274, 326]. The acyl chains of bacterial membranes may contain branches (Gram-positive bacteria) or cyclopropane rings (Gram-negative bacteria) [88].

Lipopolysaccharides (LPS)

Lipopolysaccharides (LPS) are an abundant surface component of the outer membrane of Gram-negative bacteria. Also termed endotoxins, they form a family of toxic phosphorylated glycolipids found in the outer membrane of Gram-negative bacteria, including *Campylobacter* spp., and are essential for the physical integrity and functioning of that membrane. The LPS molecule consists of three distinct regions. Anchored in the outer membrane is the lipid A moiety, which is the endotoxic part of the LPS molecule. Attached to the lipid A is the core, which consists of an inner and outer part. Finally, the O-antigen is a polysaccharide repeat and is normally attached to the outer core. Roughly speaking, it is the hydrophilic part of the LPS, which is responsible for their serological (antigenic) qualities, and the hydrophobic part for the complex of characteristics referred to with the term endotoxicity [342]. LPS possesses potent immunomodulating and immunostimulating activities, due principally to their lipid component, lipid A; harbours binding sites for antibodies and non immunoglobulin serum factors and contributes to bacterial virulence [259]. Size and structure, especially of the hydrophilic part, may vary within a wide range according to the respective LPS.

C) Campylobacter Membrane Lipids

Fatty Acid Biosynthesis

Fatty acid biosynthesis is co-ordinately regulated with phospholipid synthesis, macromolecular synthesis and growth as part of the normal response of a bacterium to a changing environment. This response is termed the stringent response, and is orchestrated by changing levels of the alarmone, ppGpp [64].

The first committed step in fatty acid biosynthesis is catalyzed by acetyl-CoA carboxylase carboxyl transferase subunit beta (accD) that forms malonyl-CoA from acetyl-CoA [186, 317]. Malonyl CoA-acyl carrier protein transacylase (FabD) transfers the malonyl group from CoA to ACP [186, 317]. Malonyl-ACP is the first intermediate necessary for fatty acid biosynthesis. Four reactions are then required to complete each round of fatty acid elongation (fig. 2).

- 3-oxoacyl-[acyl-carrier-protein] synthase III (FabH) catalyzes the condensation of acetyl-CoA with malonyl-ACP to initiate cycles of fatty acid elongation. Its position at the beginning of the pathway suggests a regulatory role and its overexpression results in an overall shortening of the fatty acid chain-lengths [167].
- The next step is the NADPH-dependent reduction of the β-acetoacetyl-ACP to (R)-3-hydroxy-butanoyl-ACP by 3-oxoacyl-[acyl-carrier protein] reductase (FabG) [186, 317].
- The β-hydroxybutanoyl-ACP is then dehydratated to the *trans*-But-2-enoyl-ACP by (3R)-hydroxymyristoyl-[acyl carrier protein] dehydratase (FabZ) [186, 317].
- The final step in the elongation cycle is the NAD(P)H-dependent reduction of But-2-enoyl-ACP to Butyryl-ACP by a putative enoyl-[acyl-carrier-protein] reductase [NADH], FabI [186, 317].

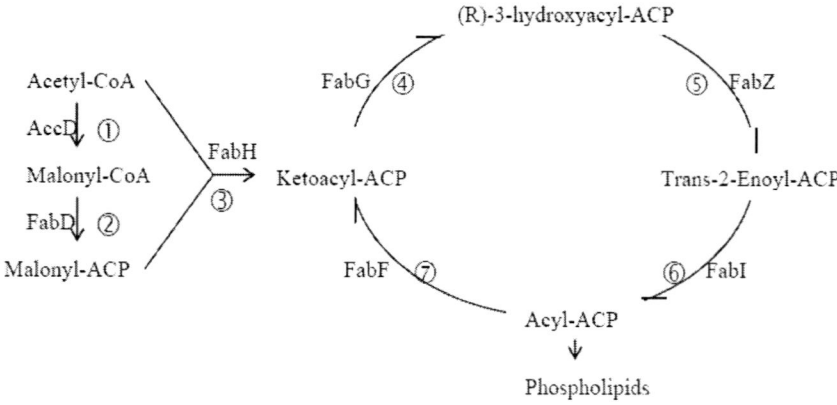

Figure 2. Schematic pathway of saturated fatty acids biosynthesis of *Campylobacter* [186, 150].

Biosynthesis of UFAs in *E. coli* occurs through the action of two key enzymes, FabA and FabB. FabA is an isoform of FabZ and differs in that FabZ catalyzes only the dehydratase reaction [256], whereas FabA is a bifunctional enzyme that also catalyses isomerization of *trans*-2-decenoyl-ACP to *cis*-3-decenoyl-ACP [135]. FabB was shown to be necessary for elongation of UFAs

[317]. The absence of *fabA* and *fabB* genes in *C. jejuni* [186] is consistent with the reported presence of these genes only in the Gram-negative α- and γ- proteobacteria.

Biosynthesis of UFAs in other bacteria may therefore occur either through a distinct pathway, or with enzymes sufficiently different not to be recognized as FabA and FabB homologues [398]. *Streptococcus pneumoniae* uses a FabM instead of FabA [236] and *Enterococcus faecalis* possesses a FabZ and a FabF with similar *E. coli* FabA and FabB functions [398]. *Bacillus subtilis* has two FabH homologs with uncommon substrate specificity, enabling synthesis of branched fatty acids. To date, the pathway of UFA biosynthesis in *Campylobacter* is still misunderstood. The presence of two FabH homologues is worthy to be noticed [336].

Bacterial cyclopropane Fatty Acids (CFA) typically appear rather abruptly at a particular stage in the growth of batch cultures [133] with a concomitant decrease of their structurally homologous UFAs [79]. The methylene addition on the *cis*-double bond by a cyclopropane synthase, occurs through the reaction of *S*-adenosylmethionine (AdoMet) with full-length UFA esterified to phospholipid. Palmitoleic (*cis*-9-hexadecenoic acid) and *cis*-vaccenic (*cis*-11-octadecenoic acid) acids are respectively the precursors of *cis*- 9, 10-methylene hexadecanoic (17:0 cyc) and *cis*-11, 12-methylene octadecanoic acids (lactobacillic acid, 19:0 cyc), both found in *Campylobacter* [336, 133, 395].

Fatty acids profiles

The determination of whole bacterial cells fatty acid profiles was used as a bacterial typing and identification method [75, 158, 204, 261, 357].

The composition of 368 strains of *Campylobacter* and *Campylobacter*-like species (CLO) was determined by Lambert *et al.* (1987), which enabled their division into seven groups [204]. All of the *Campylobacter* strains and CLO tested were found to contain tetradecanoic acid (14:0), hexadecanoic acid (16:0), octadecenoic acid (18:1 ω7-cis), and octadecanoic acid (18:0). Groups A, B, and C represented most strains (92%). Group A contained *Campylobacter jejuni* (97%) and most *C. coli* (83%) strains and was characterized by the presence of 19:0 cyc and 3-hydroxytetradecanoic (3-OH-14:0) acids. Group B includes all *C. laridis* and some *C. coli* strains and differs from group A by the absence of 19:0 cyc and the greater relative concentration of 18:1 ω7-cis. Group C contained *C. fetus* strains and was characterized by the presence of 3-OH-14:0 and hexadecanoic acids (3-OH-16:0) and the absence of 19:0 cyc. The remaining 29 strains were placed into four additional groups including *C. cinaedi*, *C. fennelliae* and *C. pyloridis*.

Recently, a computer-operated automated system for microbial identification based on the composition of cellular fatty acids [249] was built and applied by Hinton *et al.* (2004) to monitor transmission of *Campylobacter* during commercial poultry processing [158]. Dendrograms generated from fatty acid methyl ester profiles of the *Campylobacter* isolates determined the degree of relatedness between isolates recovered from carcass rinsates and scald water.

Lipopolysaccharides

Lipopolysaccharide (LPS) is considered an important virulence factor of *C. jejuni* and of many other pathogenic Gram-negative bacteria [119]. *C. jejuni* strains synthesize LPS molecules with or without an O-antigen-like repeat structure. Briefly, the basic structure comprises a lipid A moiety fairly typical of *Enterobacteriaceae*, with a fatty acid-linked and phosphorylated glucosamine or diaminoglucose disaccharide [258] to which is linked the inner core polysaccharide. LPS molecules of *Campylobacter* were shown to have endotoxic properties [267], to be involved in adherence [245] and presumably to play a role in antigenic variation, as these bacteria have the ability to shift the LPS antigenic composition [251]. The sugar composition and structure of the core oligosaccharide from several *C. jejuni* strains, belonging to eight serotypes, have been analyzed [18, 334]. *N*-acetylneuraminic acid (sialic acid), a molecule not frequently found in prokaryotes, when attached by 2-3 linkages to β-D-galactosidase, was found to look like gangliosides in structure [17]. This molecular mimicry between *Campylobacter* glycoconjugates and peripheral nerve gangliosides is thought to play a role in the neuropathological autoimmune diseases Guillain-Barré syndrome (GBS) and Miller-Fisher syndrome (MFS) [334, 339].

4.1.2. Influence of Environmental Factors on Campylobacter Membrane Lipid Composition

A) General Aspects

Alteration of bacterial membrane fluidity and lipid composition in response to environmental factors has been dealt in numerous papers. Most external factors studied in literature include temperature, pH, chemicals (pollutants, bacteriocines, *etc.*), ions (salinity inducing osmotic stress, *etc.*), pressure, nutrients and the growth phase of the microbial culture. It emerges from these studies that the basic adaptation mechanisms are similar in widely different cell types [332]. Bacterial membrane fluidity can be adjusted by the alteration of phospholipid polar head groups. However, it happens less commonly than fatty acyl chain alteration, as the former is less effective in modifying lipid fluidity or the transition temperature [324]. Regulation of bacterial membrane fluidity mostly occurs through (1) modification of saturation, (2) isomerisation *cis* to *trans* unsaturation [151], (3) branching and cyclisation [332, 367, 396], and (4) elongation of fatty acids [332].

B) Influence of Temperature on Campylobacter Membrane Lipid Composition

Influence of Temperature on Transition from Spiral to Coccoid Forms

Temperature is known to affect significantly the content and composition of microbial lipids (see [326] for a review). The phase transition of lipids from the crystalline to the liquid-crystalline form has been found to occur outside their growth temperature range [146]. An increase in the level of unsaturation and a decrease in the average chain length of the fatty acids as growth temperature decreases is often observed [327, 326]. Influence of temperature on the fatty acid composition of *Campylobacter jejuni* during transition from spiral to coccoid form was studied by Hazeleger *et al.* (1995) [147]. Stationary *C. jejuni* cells were incubated at different low temperatures (4 – 12 and 25°C) in order to show if a correlation could be drawn between the cell form (spiral or coccoid) and the fatty acid profile. Membrane fatty acid composition of cocci formed at low temperatures was found to be almost identical to that of spiral cells, whereas that of cocci formed at 25°C was clearly different. The significant increase in the amount of hexadecanoic and octadecanoic acids and the decreased concentration of tetradecanoic, hexadecenoic and 19-cyclopropane acids observed in cocci formed at 25°C, showed that the fatty acid composition of cocci was strongly influenced by the temperature at which cocci were formed.

Adaptation of Campylobacter to Suboptimal Temperatures

Höller *et al.* (1998) determined *Campylobacter coli* fatty acid profiles following incubation of cells in Schaedler broth in the dark at 4 – 10 – 20 and 37°C [160]. Stress due to low temperatures, *i.e.*, 20°C, altered *C. coli* fatty acid pattern dramatically, although the bacteria is not able to grow at this temperature.

An increase in the short-chain and unsaturated acids was noted; above all, a drastic increase in 19:0 cyc with a concomitant decrease of 18:1, its precursor, was observed at 20°C. At 37°C, no effect was noticed on the 19:0 cyc concentration. Höller et al. correlated the increase in short-chain, unsaturated and cyclopropane fatty acids with the decrease of membrane fluidity induced by low temperature. Citing Leach et al. [206] and Hazeleger et al. [147], they underlined the complex role of 19:0 cyc which was attributed by the former to general reaction to stress whereas the experiments conducted at different low temperatures by the latter led to different and unexplainable results.

C) Influence of the Growth Parameters on Campylobacter Membrane

Lipid Composition

Influence of Growth Rate

Leach et al. (1997) described the influence of the growth rate on the membrane lipid composition of *C. jejuni* in continuous cultures [206]. The substitution patterns of phospholipids were found to depend on growth rate. In particular, the proportion of cyclopropane (19:0 cyc) substituted species was shown to increase at the expense of the corresponding 18:1 precursors at low growth rate maintained by low dilution rate. Leach et al. hypothetized that the proportion of *C. jejuni* cyclopropane fatty acids might increase similarly to those of *Escherichia coli, Streptococcus lactis* and *Vibrio cholerae* in late logarithmic and stationary phase [396] or when cells are exposed to stresses such as pH, high temperature [78] or starvation [134]. The formation of 19:0 cyc in *E. coli* is performed by a soluble, *in vivo* unstable, cytoplasmic cyclopropane fatty acid (CFA) synthase which synthesis is growth phase-dependent. In *E. coli, cfa* gene is transcribed from two promoters, one of them being active only during the log-to-stationary phase transition and depending on the putative sigma factor (*rpoS (katF)*). It results in a large increase in the CFA synthase activity during the log-to-stationary phase transition although the enzyme is synthesized throughout the growth curve [396]. The genome analysis actually revealed the presence of a cyclopropane-fatty-acyl-phospholipid synthase [336, 294]. However *C. jejuni* is unusual in lacking sigma factor S, σ^S, or any other sigma factor associated with stationary phase adaptation, which could account for the large increase in the CFA synthase activity during the log-to-stationary phase transition [291, 294].

Influence of Growth Phase

Martinez-Rodriguez and Mackey (2005) observed that *C. jejuni* cells were more resistant to high hydrostatic pressure than those in exponential phase [240]. This was unexpected given the reported lack of any similar changes in resistance to heat, acid and oxidative stress [189, 264], but indicated that at least some physiological changes occurred in stationary phase. Changes in *C. jejuni* membrane fatty acid composition during growth were recorded to understand the greater high-pressure resistance of *C. jejuni* cells as they passed from active growth to stationary phase. As growth progressed, a large decrease in the membrane content of UFAs (16:1 and 18:1) and a corresponding increase in 17:0 and 19:0 cyclopropane fatty acids were observed. There was also a noticeable increase in short chain fatty acids (12:0 and 14:0) and a slight decrease in saturated fatty acids (16:0 and 18:0). The stationary phase membrane changes in *C. jejuni,* particularly the characteristic increase in cyclopropane fatty acids were similar to those reported in other Gram-negative bacteria. The authors mentioned that the cyclopropane fatty acid protective effect observed in *E. coli* against freezing damage, exposure to ethanol and much more against acid stress [49, 67, 132] could not be asserted in *C. jejuni* [264]considering their little role in acid resistance. However these changes may represent a general response to changes in growth rate or exposure to stress, rather than being specific to stationary phase and this will require further investigation.

Conclusion

The atypical stress response of *C. jejuni* makes the interpretation of physiological alterations difficult. The membrane directly in contact with the environment is a privileged target of these stresses. To date, biosynthetic pathways of *Campylobacter* unsaturated and cyclopropane fatty acids are unclear. Moreover, the role of cyclopropane fatty acids is misunderstood, resulting in contradictory interpretations. More research is needed to understand how *Campylobacter* counteracts the modifications of its environment and to know if alteration of membrane fluidity is involved in its survival strategy.

4.2. Membrane and Antimicrobial Resistance in *Campylobacter* SPP

Introduction

The outer cell layer of Gram-negative bacteria consists of an outer membrane (OM), a thin layer of peptidoglycan and a periplasmic space located between the outer membrane and the peptidoglycan/cytoplasmic membrane (fig. 3). The OM composition (phospholipids and lipopolysaccharide (LPS)) renders it impermeable to many substrates. Channel-forming proteins, in particular non-specific ones called porins, are therefore also present in the OM to enable the influx of hydrophilic compounds.

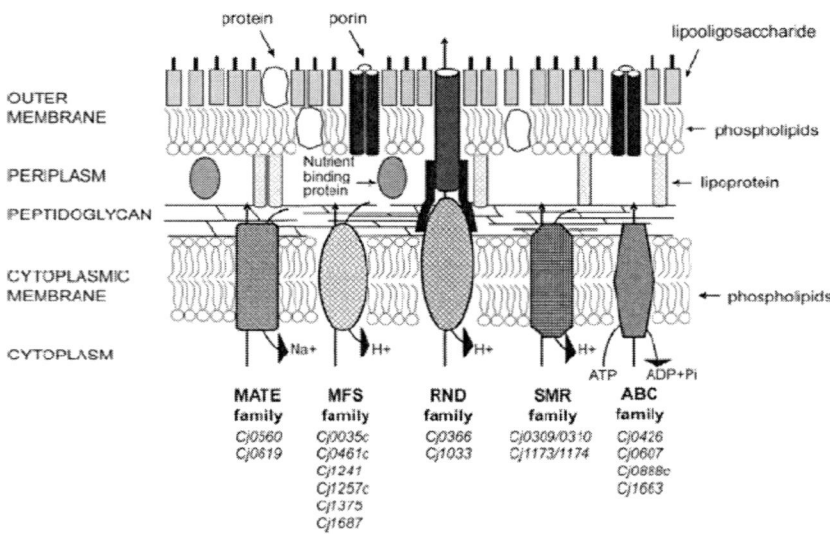

Figure 3. Structure and composition of the membrane in *Campylobacter* spp, including lipooligosaccharide, porins and the five families of transporters (major facilitator superfamily (MFS), ATP-binding cassette (ABC) family, resistance-nodulation-division (RND) family, small multidrug resistance (SMR) family and multidrug and toxic compound extrusion (MATE) family) detailed in the text. Below each family of transporters are indicated the homologs found in the sequenced genome of *C. jejuni* NCTC 11168.

Transport of Drugs through the Membrane and Antimicrobial Resistance

The principal targets of antimicrobials are located in the cytoplasm or in the cytoplasmic membrane. Drugs thus need to be transported across the outer membrane to reach their target. Depending on their chemical structure, drugs can employ the porin pathway (e.g. hydrophilic molecules such as beta-lactams or fluoroquinolones), diffuse through the lipid bilayer (e.g. macrolides) or employ a self-promoted uptake (e.g. aminoglycosides).

Apart from specific resistance mechanisms (target mutation or modification, drug inactivation and metabolic shunt), bacteria can achieve drug resistance by limiting the amount of drug that enters the cell (OM permeability) or by actively effluxing antimicrobials that reach the cytoplasm.

Campylobacter spp., in particular *C. jejuni* and *C. coli*, are intrinsically resistant to a number of antibiotics including bacitracin, novobiocin, rifampin, trimethoprim, vancomycin and usually also cephalothin [375]. All these resistance mechanisms have not been elucidated but many of them probably involve the inability of the drugs to penetrate the cells. In addition, acquired resistance to many antibiotics (ampicillin, chloramphenicol, macrolides, aminoglycosides, tetracyclines and quinolones) has been described in *Campylobacter* spp. [375]. Most of the resistance mechanisms examined involve drug inactivation (aminoglycoside phosphotransferase or nucleotidyltransferase, beta-lactamase, chloramphenicol acetyltransferase) or target protection (*tetO* determinant of tetracycline resistance) [375] but increased efflux of some antimicrobials has also been described [217] and many resistance mechanisms have not been characterized yet.

LPS and Antimicrobial Resistance

LPS is largely responsible for the impermeability of the bilayer to hydrophobic molecules [386]. LPS is composed of lipid A, a core polysaccharide and the O-antigen. Saturation of the fatty acid substituents leads to a low fluidity of the OM. In addition, the highly negatively charged O-antigen and the cross-bridging of the core region via phosphate groups and divalent cations also contribute to the low permeability of the LPS [277].

Campylobacter spp., as *Neisseria* spp. and *Haemophilus influenzae*, do not carry an O-antigen on their LPS (thus renamed LOS for lipooligosaccharide) [259] (fig. 3). This could explain the greater susceptibility of these Gram-negative pathogens to the hydrophobic macrolide molecules. Molecules of LPS with a high molecular weight have been described in *Campylobacter* suggesting the existence of a 'smooth' phenotype in some strains but these structures seem to be capsular [185].

The composition of LOS is highly variable in *Campylobacter* due to frequent intergenomic recombinations and to a phase variation in the genes encoding LOS biosynthesis [185]. This variability could have an impact on the OM hydrophobicity and thus on diffusion of drugs across the OM membrane but this has not been examined yet in this bacterium.

Porins and Antimicrobial Resistance

Antibiotics such as beta-lactams, chloramphenicol and fluoroquinolones permeate the outer membrane via porins. Changes in the number of porin molecules, size or selectivity will alter the rate of diffusion of these antibiotics.

Examples of antibiotic resistance (in particular fluoroquinolone resistance) resulting from a downregulation of porin expression have been described in several bacteria including S*erratia marcescens*, *Escherichia coli*, *Salmonella enterica*, *H. influenzae*, *Klebsiella pneumoniae* and *Enterobacter aerogenes* [199]. This usually leads to a low-level resistance which combined with other mechanisms of resistance. In several bacteria, loss of porins appeared to be indirectly regulated by the *mar* operon, which controlled the expression of at least 60 genes including genes encoding multidrug efflux systems. Porin expression was also influenced by different growth conditions including temperature, osmolarity and pH but also by structural factors such as LPS and chaperone proteins [286].

Expression of porins with different pore selectivity has also been reported in *E. coli*, with the OmpC porin (low pore diameter) being expressed at high temperature and high osmolarity on the contrary of the OmpF porin (higher pore diameter) expressed at low temperature or low osmolarity.

Cases of resistance resulting from a sequence modification of porins have also been described in several bacteria. Mutation in the primary sequence resulted in a constriction of the channel formed by the encoded porin protein, which modified the drug selectivity of the pore [286].

In *Campylobacter*, two porins have been described: a major outer membrane protein (MOMP) [39, 82] and a minor one: Omp50 [40] which appears to be specific of *C. jejuni* [86]. The MOMP belongs to the family of trimeric porins and showed two distinct functional structures: one trimeric and one monomeric with both cation selectivity [82]. LPS could play an important role in assembling the porin trimers. Expression of the MOMP protein was found to increase with temperature and pH [85]. No correlation between porin modification or modification of porin expression and antibiotic resistance has been observed yet in *Campylobacter* [227, 295]. However, an atypical quinolone resistance pattern (ciprofloxacin resistance but nalidixic susceptibility) has been described in an isolate of *Campylobacter jejuni* [20]. The resistance mechanism has not been elucidated. One hypothesis could be that a modification of membrane permeability (porin modification for example), which differentially impacts on the two molecules, could have occurred in this isolate (amphoteric and hydrophilic characteristics of fluoroquinolone favor the porin pathway of entry, whereas hydrophobic characteristics and negative charge of nalidixic acid would rather favor the diffusion pathway).

Efflux Systems Involved in Antimicrobial Resistance in Campylobacter

Most of the Gram-negative bacteria are more resistant to antibiotics than Gram-positive bacteria. The presence of an efficient outer membrane barrier could not be the sole explanation since it could not avoid diffusion of molecules and establishment of equilibrium between outside and inside drug concentration. This is rather due to cooperation between the outer membrane barrier and efflux of the antibiotic.

Bacterial efflux systems belong to five classes: the major facilitator superfamily (MFS), the ATP-binding cassette (ABC) family, the resistance-nodulation-division (RND) family, the small multidrug resistance (SMR) family and the multidrug and toxic compound extrusion (MATE) family [304] (fig. 3). RND transporters form a tripartite system, including a periplasmic membrane fusion protein (MFP) and an outer membrane protein (fig. 3). This organization can also be seen with ABC transporter (e.g. the macrolide-specific MacAB-TolC efflux system of *E. coli*) and MF exporter (e.g. the VceAB multidrug efflux system of *Vibrio cholerae*). Drug efflux systems can be drug/class specific or capable of accommodating diverse chemically distinct substrates.

Lin et al. [215] and Pumbwe and Piddock [307] both described the first efflux system in *Campylobacter jejuni* (CmeABC), conferring intrinsic resistance to multiple antibiotics (including fluoroquinolones, erythromycin, ampicillin, tetracycline, chloramphenicol), detergents and dyes. The CmeB protein is structurally and functionally similar to members of the RND superfamily of transporters described in other Gram negative bacterial pathogens. The *cmeABC* operon is widely distributed in different *Campylobacter* strains, including *C. coli* [56, 76] and is constitutively expressed in wild-type strains [215, 216, 295]. Expression of the CmeABC efflux pump is controlled by the CmeR transcriptional regulator, which belongs to the TetR family of repressors [217]. An insertional *cmeR* mutant of the 81-176 *C. jejuni* strain exhibited a higher resistance level to low concentrations of ciprofloxacin and this correlated with the overexpression of the CmeABC pump components [217]. A similar correlation was observed in a multidrug resistant mutant of the same strain, obtained after selection on increasing amounts of ciprofloxacin [217]. This mutant contained a single nucleotide deletion in the binding region of CmeR located in the promoter region of the *cmeABC* operon [217]. We also recently described an *in vitro*-selected multidrug resistant isolate carrying a point mutation in the binding site of the CmeR protein, which decreased the affinity of the repressor [57]. Pumbwe et al [308] measured the expression of the *cmeB* gene in multidrug resistant isolates of *C. jejuni* and found that one third of the isolates overexpressed the *cmeB* gene. These isolates accumulated l ciprofloxacin. The CmeABC efflux pump functions synergically with 23S rRNA mutations to confer a high level of resistance to erythromycin and with a Thr86Ile modification in the GyrA subunit to confer fluoroquinolone resistance [297]. It is also responsible for low-level macrolide resistance in *C. jejuni* and *C. coli* [56, 230, 232, 296] and is essential for *Campylobacter* colonization of intestinal tract of chickens by mediating bile salt resistance [217-219, 216]. Inhibition of this pump may prevent the emergence of fluoroquinolone- and erythromycin-resistant mutants of *Campylobacter* [238, 310, 411]. Analysis of the sequenced genomes of *Campylobacter* revealed only two homologues of activators of efflux systems (one homolog of BltR of *Bacillus subtilis* and one homolog of Rob of *E. coli*, with 24 and 25 % of identity respectively). Homologs of the global regulators of efflux systems (MarA, SoxS, RamA) found in other bacteria are missing in *Campylobacter*. Analysis of the promoter region of the *cmeABC* operon revealed a 17 pb-spacing between the -35 and -10 boxes (localized 60 pb upstream of the start codon of the *cmeA* gene and 14 pb upstream the binding site of the CmeR repressor) and a degenerated Rob-box upstream the -35 box (Cagliero C. and Payot S., *unpublished results*). It would be worth examining the implication of the Rob homolog (Cj1042 in the NCTC 11168 strain) in the regulation of the CmeABC efflux system.

A second efflux pump, CmeDEF, was described in *Campylobacter jejuni* [309]. Insertional mutagenesis of *cmeF* in the NCTC 11168 strain only resulted in modest changes in the susceptibility to a few antimicrobials (ampicillin, deoxycholate, triclosan, cetrimide), while the *cmeF* mutation in *C. jejuni* 81-176 did not change its susceptibility to ciprofloxacin, erythromycin, tetracycline, and chloramphenicol. CmeDEF seems to interact with CmeABC in conferring antimicrobial resistance and maintaining cell viability in *C. jejuni* [6]. *cmeDEF* is regulated by a transcriptional factor, but the identity of the regulator and the impact of overexpression of this system in respect of resistance to antimicrobials in *Campylobacter* remain to be determined.

In vitro exposition of *cmeB* and *cmeF* insertional mutants to increasing concentrations of ciprofloxacin led to multidrug resistant mutants that expressed the *cmeB* and *cmeF* genes at the same levels compared to original genetic backgrounds used for selection. This observation suggested the involvement of another efflux pump or a reduced uptake of these antibiotics [309]. In addition, Mamelli et al [232, 231] and Lin et al [219] showed that an efflux pump inhibitor was still efficient in *cmeB* mutants and suggested that another efflux pump was active in *Campylobacter*.

Many other genes encoding putative efflux systems of the different families of transporters (MFS, SMR, ABC and MATE) are present in the sequenced genomes of *C. jejuni* NCTC 11168 and RM1221 and *C. coli* RM 2228. Ge et al [125] inactivated genes encoding 8 putative efflux pumps (4, 2 and 2 homologs of the MFS, MATE and SMR families of transporters respectively) in addition to the *cmeB* and *cmeF* genes. They found that, except for the *cmeB* gene, inactivation of the genes encoding these putative efflux pumps has no effect on susceptibility to chloramphenicol, ciprofloxacin, erythromycin and tetracycline. Recently, we inactivated the gene coding for a homolog of the ABC transporter MacB of *E. coli* [195] and *Salmonella* [280] (Cj0607, 43-44% of identity in amino acids) in wild-type and *cmeB* mutants of various strains of *C. jejuni* and *C. coli*. We did not find any change in the susceptibility of the single or double mutants to various antimicrobials (Cagliero C. and Payot S., *unpublished results*). The role of these putative efflux systems in antimicrobial resistance of *Campylobacter* thus needs further investigation.

Conclusion

Membrane of the bacteria constitutes the first barrier to the efficacy of drugs and several components of the membrane can be modified by the bacteria to counter the adverse effects of antibiotics.

Modifications of LPS and porins have been described as mechanisms of antimicrobial resistance in several bacteria. In *Campylobacter*, a link between LPS and antimicrobial resistance has not been described yet. No correlation has been established between modification of porin or of porin expression and antimicrobial resistance either. However, two membrane efflux systems CmeABC and CmeDEF have been described and play a role in antimicrobial resistance in *Campylobacter*. There is also evidence that other efflux systems are active in this bacterium and characterization of the other putative transporters is needed, as well as an understanding of the regulation of efflux systems since it differs from other previously studied bacteria.

4.3. *C. jejuni* Senses Its Environment by Two-Component Systems (TCS)

The ability to respond quickly to changes in the environment is essential for the success of the bacterium and requires it to be able to sense its surroundings and modify its physiology accordingly. Over a decade ago, the term « two component » was used to describe a new class of regulatory systems found in bacteria. Two-component systems serve as a basic stimulus-response coupling mechanism to allow organisms to sense and respond to changes in many different environmental conditions. The system comprise a cytoplasmic membrane-associated histidine protein kinase (HK), containing a conserved kinase core, and a response regulator protein (RR), containing a conserved regulatory domain. Extracellular stimuli are sensed by and serve to modulate the activities of the HK. The HK tranfers a phosphoryl group to the RR, in a reaction catalyzed by the RR. Phosphotransfer to the RR results in activation of a downstream effector domain that elicits the specific response [362]. There seems to be a correlation between the number of these systems and the ability of bacteria to adapt to environmental conditions. In fact, in *B. subtilis*, which can exist in and tolerate a wide range of environments there are 70 encoding RRs [104]. In *E. coli* there are 30 HKs and 32 RRs. In contrast, *H. pylori*, which occupies only a limited number of environment niches, contains just 4 sensor proteins and 7 RRs [362]. Analysis of the genome sequence of *C. jejuni* revealed the presence of 11 putative response regulators, six histidine sensor proteins and one hybrid sensor response regulator protein [294]. Six of the genes encoding *C. jejuni* response regulators, have been characterized to date. Five of the six TCSs in *Campylobacter* spp. are involved in colonization. The RacR-RacS system (Reduced ability to colonize) is important for growth and avian intestine colonization [46]. The CbrR system (*Campylobacter* bile resistant) modulates sodium deoxycholate resistance and chicken colonization [312]. FlgR is involved in the Fla regulon. The chicken colonization rate of a *Campylobacter* FlgR mutant is strongly reduced even if Wösten *et al.* 2004 suggested that this FlgR (Flagellar genes) mutant behaviour is essentially caused via its effect on flagella expression [407]. The two-component signal transduction system (Cj1222c-Cj1223c) has been designated as dccR-dccS for diminished capacity to colonize. Although *C. jejuni* mutants defective for the DccRS system grew and survived identically to wild type under *in vitro* growth conditions but they exhibited a reduction of colonization in animal models [228]. The CheA-CheY (see chemotaxis paragraph), has been demonstrated by Yao *et al.* (1997) as involved in virulence [412]. A CheY mutant resulted in a hyperadherent and hyperinvasive phenotype, but was unable to colonize mice or cause disease in ferrets. In the only case of PhosR-PhosS system involved in the phosphate regulon and recently described, the colonization behaviour of the phoR mutant remained similar to the wild type [406].

4.4. Motility, Chemotaxis

Studies about colonization have shown that *Campylobacter* was able to actively swimm up and down in the intestinal crypts [207].The production of flagella and flagellar motility are important determinants of *C. jejuni* for pathogenic interactions with various hosts. *Campylobacters* produce a single flagellum at one or both poles of the bacterium. As in enteric group bacteria, the *C. jejuni* flagellum comprises three structural elements : basal body, hook and filament. The majority of genes involved in biogenesis of this complex structure, a total of about 40, are conserved with those of the well-defined paradigm based on research in *E. coli* [229]. The filament of the flagellum which is the major part of the complex has been the first and the most intensively studied domain. It is probably due to the characterization of the flagellins as the first antigens of *C.*

jejuni and *C.coli* [270]. Consequently, in complement to the genotyping methods which produce information about the basic framework of a strain, various techniques (PCR-RFLP, DGGE or MLST) employed for flagellin genes typing have been developed to focus on these particular loci. Contrary to *E. coli*, the filament of *C. jejuni* is composed of two different flagellins named FlaA and FlaB. Surprisingly, the comparison of the two protein sequences of FlaA and FlaB deduced from DNA reveals a lot of similarities and only few variations in their central region. Mutants in FlaA were poorly motile and possessed only short truncated flagella, while mutants in FlaB possessed near-normal flagella and motility but in some experiments showed some decrease in the pathogenic potential [136, 400]. The conclusion was that FlaA was the major flagellin while FlaB was a minor component of the flagella [400]. More recently studies have shown that over-expression of FlaB could compensate the FlaA deletion, indicating that there are complexities in flagellin expression that are not yet fully understood [140]. Even if many genes of the flagellar structure are similar to the *E. coli* or *Salmonella* paradigm, their regulation of expression differs significantly. Recent studies have shown that *C. jejuni* possesses two alternative σ factors, σ^{28} and σ^{54}, to mediate transcriptional regulation of specific flagellar genes [63, 153, 154, 407]. It is the main difference with the enteric group paradigm system of regulation, where there is no known involvement of σ^{54} in the flagellar gene expression [171]. In *C. jejuni*, σ^{28} is thightly involved in the transcription of the FlaA and a few additional flagellar genes, while σ^{54} is implicated in a more global cascade of genes regulation encoding the flagellar rod, basal body, hook components and a minor flagellin. σ^{54} mutants showed complete absence of flagella and flagellin expression while σ^{28} mutants revealed truncated flagella and partial flagellin expression [170]. Previous studies have shown that activation transcription of σ^{54}–dependent flagellar genes is dependent on the FlgSR two-component system and the proteins of the flagellar export apparatus, including FlhA, FlhB, FliP and FliR [154]. These authors have proposed that these two systems may constitute a regulatory cascade where the formation of export flagellar apparatus and/or the secretory activity of the flagellum may activate the FlgS sensor kinase. Then FlgS could phosphorylate the FlgR σ^{54} –dependent response regulator, activating it for transcription of σ^{54} – dependent flagellar genes [407]. FlgR like transcriptional activator is frequently found in polar flagellated bacteria such as *Vibrio cholerae* [306], *Pseudomonas aeroginosa* [16] or *Helicobacter pylori* [353]. But very recently, Sommerlad and Hendrixson (2007), have described FlgP and FlgQ necessary required for motility but whose expression would be independent on σ^{28} and σ^{54}, suggesting an other way of regulation unknown uptoday [351].

Depending on the environmental conditions (especially *in vitro*) flagellated and aflagellated phenotypes have been observed in *C. jejuni*. This ability of some strains to turn on or off the expression of flagella has been termed phase variation [59]. Jones *et al.* (1993) have shown that this motility could be restored by passage *in vivo* through the avian intestinal tract or selected *in vitro* by special media [184]. A study of Hendrixson (2006) suggests that this phase variation results from generation of variants due to the presence of hypervariable sequences composed of short homopolymeric runs of nucleotides in the particular locus of FlgR. In fact, this phase variation could generate, *in vivo*, aflagellated cells less fit for colonization and then shed into the environment via the faecal matter. This phase variation is now explored as a mechanism *in vivo* to promote successful transmission to new host where these individuals variants may revert a flagellated phenotype able to colonize [155].

Table 10. Comparaison of chemotaxis proteins present in *E. coli*, *B. subtilis* and *C. jejuni*

Gene Product	Activity	E. coli	B. subtilis	C. jejuni
CheA	Histidine kinase	+	+	+ (CheAY)
CheB	Methyl esterase	+	+	+
CheC	Phosphatase and additional protein	-	+	-
CheD	Glutamine deamidase	-	+	-
CheR	Methyl transferase	+	+	+
CheV	Coupling and additional protein	-	+	+
CheW	Coupling protein	+	+	+
CheY	Response regulator	+	+	+
CheZ	Phosphatase	+	-	-
FliY	Phosphatase at the flagellar switch	-	+	+

Chemotaxis proteins could be separated in three different functions: signal recognition/transduction, excitation, adaptation/signal removal.

Given that Campylobacters are able of movements which confer advantages to this organism in the colonization process of intestinal tracts, the following paragraph summarizes the chemotaxis mechanism involved in the transmission of a signal of changes in the environment to the flagellar motor. The chemotaxis is the most studied of all the signal transduction systems that control movement of bacteria. Hugdhal *et al.* (1988) have demonstrated the chemotaxis capacities of *Campylobacter jejuni* with different chemoattractants as mucin, pyruvate and succinate [162]. While the motility apparatus differs among bacteria, the general control mechanism is conserved throughout all the bacteria and archaea [368]. However, the genome study of *Campylobacter* revealed homologies and differences with *E. coli* and *B. subtilis* which are summarized in table 10.

Signal Recognition/Transduction

Sensing of chemoattractants or chemorepellents is mediated by methyl-accepting chemotaxis proteins (MCP) present in the periplasmic domain. In the genome study of *Campylobacter jejuni*, 10 potential chemotaxis receptors (designated Tlp for transducer-like protein) which may bind ligands have been identified [294]. A first group of these receptors have a similar structure of MCP proteins characterized in *E. coli* however it remains impossible to determine which receptors are directly involved in a particular monitoring of the periplasmic environment. A second group of three genes (Cj1191c-1189c) named respectively, *aer1*, *cetA* for (*Campylobacter* energy taxis) and *cetB* or *aer2*, were alternatively described as required for energy and aerotaxis system even if the exact role of *aer1* for instance, which does not affect motility remains unknown [153]. A third group which is similar to family C transducers in *H.salinarum* [414], contains receptor proteins which detect modification in the cytoplasmic domain and thus sense the internal physiological changes.

Excitation

Contrary to the chemosensory complex diversity, the excitation domain is very conserved throughout all bacteria. The centerpiece of the chemotaxis system is a two-component system name CheA kinase that autophosphorylates and passes the phosphate group onto CheY response regulator. In *Campylobacter* the CheA domain (Cj0284) is fused to a C-terminal RR domain corresponding to a CheAY hybrid system. A paraloguous sequence of CheY has been found elsewhere in the chromosome (Cj1118) [294]. CheY response regulator governs the clockwise of flagellar rotation by an interaction with the flagellar motor. Marchant *et al.* (1998) verified in *C. jejuni* that the CheY mutant cells were motile with a straight swimming and were not able to change direction [234]. Two other proteins CheW and CheV are present in *C. jejuni* and complexed with the CheA structure. CheW has no regulatory function but an essential role for the formation of the ternary complex which permits the excitation process [15]. This protein is absent from the *E. coli* genome but present in *H. pylori* and *B. subtilis*. CheV is a fusion protein between CheW and CheY response regulator and its role in motility has been already experimentally demonstrated [153].

Adaptation/Signal Removal

As mentioned in table 10, many proteins are involved in the adaptation system. To sense higher concentrations of attractants or to modify the bacterial motion when the bacterium is moving in a wrong direction, the system has to be able to adaptation. In *E. coli*, this adaptation is only methylation dependent. The activity of CheB (a methylesterase) is activated when the amino-terminal RR domain of CheB is phosphorylated by P-CheA [368]. The demethylation of the MCP receptors by CheB acts as a feedback loop. But when comparing the *C. jejuni* CheB sequence with the one of *E. coli* for instance, the main difference is the absence of a RR domain in the CheB of *C. jejuni*. Its function is thus predicted as the stabilization of the active sites of methylation by a complex formation with CheR a methyltransferase. Interestingly, in *B. subtilis*, the CheV RR domain is thought to have a function in methylation [321]. Thus in *C. jejuni* CheV could have the same function and inhibit CheB directly or its access to the methylation sites. A second way of action could be the direct modulation of the CheA kinase activity by a modification in the conformation of the ternary complex [235] to remove or adapt the signal.

4.5. Biofilms

Biofilms have been defined initially as 'cells immobilized at a substratum and frequently embedded in an organic polymer matrix of microbial origin' [68]. This definition was afterwards completed by Costerton *et al.* [77] indicating that biofilms consist in a 'matrix-enclosed bacterial populations adherent to each other and/or to surfaces or interfaces'. Although biofilm formation is a continuous process, three steps could be distinguished: (i) cell attachment, (ii) cell proliferation, and (iii) cell maturation. The former step could be divided into two phases: the reversible cell attachment and the irreversible cell attachment and the latter step could refer to the life of the biofilm with growth and erosion or sloughing phases. The cells or the microcolonies developed in the biofilm are subjected to biofilm environment composed of an extracellular matrix of exopolymeric substances amended with free molecules finding in the liquid phase and water channels that allow nutrients, waste, and gas to circulate through the biofilm. The term 'sessile' is usually attributed to the cells embedded in the matrix and the term 'planktonic' usually refers to free cell counterparts. The position of the cells inside the biofilm would determine their mode of growth (from sessile to planktonic cells) and their metabolic activity (from dormant to highly active state). The biofilm could be composed of various bacterial species (multi-species biofilm) or a single bacterial species (mono-species biofilm).

Campylobacter in Multi-Species Biofilm

A *Campylobacter* outbreak in 1984 caused by the contamination of chickens on a broiler farm during 18 months in southern England originated from contaminated water supply system [298]. Although no *Campylobacter* was isolated by conventional culturing methods, examination of the biofilm developed inside the water supply system revealed the presence of clumps of *Campylobacter* detected using fluorescent-antibody methods. This finding indicated that *Campylobacter* could survive into biofilms developed in the water supply systems as viable but not cultivable form (VBNC). Studies conducted on the VBNC state of *Campylobacter* cells revealed that this pathogen switches on a VBNC state when it is submitted to adverse environmental conditions [205, 378] and when the cells are organized in biofilm [99, 335, 383]. Lehtola *et al.* [212] found that *C. jejuni* could survive at least one week in a biofilm composed of indigeneous bacteria present in drinking water whereas no more planktonic *C. jejuni* could be detected after one day in the drinking water. The study indicated also that *C. jejuni* had been released from the biofilm for at least three weeks after the inoculation. *C. jejuni* survived longer time in the presence of indigenous bacteria in drinking water than in sterile water [53, 383]. Interestingly, aerobiosis decreased the survival time by 30%, but improved the persistence time by more than threefold [53]. The biofilm containing *Campylobacter* could survive longer time at cold temperatures (42 d at 4°C) than at mild temperatures (28 d at 30°C). The presence of multi-species biofilms decreased the effectiveness of sanitizers (chlorine, quaternary ammonia, peracetic acid, and peroctanoic acid mixture) against *C. jejuni* [382]. However, trisodium phosphate (8% for 2 min) was efficient to reduce both suspended and attached *C. jejuni* on stainless steel [350].

Mono-Species Biofilm of Campylobacter

Mono-species biofilms of *C. jejuni* could exist as three forms in liquid culture at both 30°C and 37°C: (i) cells attached to inert surfaces, (ii) aggregates of cells floating in the liquid, and (iii) pellicles of cells at the liquid-gas interface [176, 179]. Joshua *et al.* [176] observed that the eight test strains of *C. jejuni*, including 11168H, had the ability to attach to glass and to form a pellicle at the gas-liquid interface but only four strains could form aggregates. *C. jejuni* could adhere and develop biofilms on nitrocellulose [179], on glass surface [176], on glass fiber [179], on glass beads (Dykes), and on stainless steel [179, 350] at 37°C or 42°C. No cell was detected on polystyrene [179], nor on buna-N rubber [350]. Biofilm reached 10^6 cfu *C. jejuni*/cm^2 after two days of incubation in nutrient broth at 42°C [350]. Thicker biofilms were exhibited on nitrocellulose membrane and glass fiber than on stainless steel surface after three days of incubation at 37°C [179]. The biofilm mode of growth into aggregates allows *C. jejuni* to survive 24 d at ambient temperature and atmosphere compared to 12 d for the planktonic counterparts. The cells attached to glass and cells in pellicular biofilm fell into aggregates after 12 d and could also survive to ambient atmospheric and temperature for several weeks [176].

Microscopic observations of *C. jejuni* biofilms using scanning electronic microscopy suggested that the biofilm structure of the three forms is composed of cells embedded in an extracellular polymeric matrix (EPM) [176, 179]. The EPM was similar for the cells attached to glass or the cells organized into aggregates with a flattened and extensive EPM whereas the connections between cells in pellicular biofilm were less flattened. In *C. jejuni* biofilms, the nature of this connecting material between cells remains unknown. In other mono-species biofilms, the EPM was frequently related to exopolysacharides and/or exoproteins. No protein associated with bacterial exopolymer synthesis was found to be overexpressed in sessile cells of *C. jejuni* [179] and the mutation in genes affecting capsular polysaccharide formation (*kps*M) or the N-linked protein glycosylation pathway (*pgl*H) did not affect the biofilm formation ability of *C. jejuni* 11168H [176]. Consequently, the capsule and the protein glycosylation process are probably not related with the EPM synthesis of *C. jejuni*. However, some proteins exhibited enhanced expression in sessile cells as compared to planktonic cells. These included proteins involved in various motility functions such as flagellins (FlaA and FlaB), the filament-associated protein (FlaG), the putative hook-associated protein (FlgK), the filament cap (FliD), two proteins that may be associated with the basal body (FlgG2 and FlgG), and the chemotaxis protein CheA [179]. The mutants affected in genes involved in the flagella synthesis (*fli*S and *maf*5) neither adhered to glass surface, nor formed pellicles, at the same level as the parental strain [176]. Inactivation of other genes involved in the flagellar synthesis (*fla*B, *fla*C, and *fla*G) and the motility system (*flh*A, *fli*A, and *fla*A) led also to a delay in the pellicle formation indicating that motility and flagellar structure are implicated in the biofilm formation of *C. jejuni* [179]. The biofilm structure related to surfaces or gas-liquid interfaces was therefore mediated by flagella. This finding is consistent with other studies demonstrating the role of flagella in the initial step of the formation of the biofilm [194, 284, 390]. A transcriptomic and a translational study on *C. jejuni* 11168 revealed also that some genes involved in the flagella synthesis (*fla*B, *flh*A, and *fli*A) are also induced in suspended cells as compared to immobilized cells growing on agar surfaces [335]. Consequently, flagella may have pleiotropic functions that could be requested alternatively according to the mode of growth of the cells. From motility function in planktonic cells, flagella could change to adhesin function in sessile cells.

Proteins contributing to the survival of the cells to adverse conditions were also upregulated in biofilms of *C. jejuni*. Among them, the alkyl hydroperoxide reductase (AhpC), required in the oxidative defence process was induced in both immobilized cells on agar and biofilms [179, 335], heat shock proteins (GroEL, GroES, ClpP, and EF-G) are also overexpressed as compared to planktonic counterparts. Proteins involved in the phosphate and molybdate-transport systems, in the iron uptake, in the scaffolding protein requested in the synthesis of Fe-S proteins, and in the ferritin transportation exhibited also enhanced expression in immobilized cells or biofilms [179, 335]. An experiment conducted on the mutation of the gene encoding the putative phosphate acetyltransferase (*Cj*0688) affected the cell attachment meaning that this enzyme is important in the biofilm formation. The biofilm formation was also affected in the *Escherichi coli* counterpart muted on the gene encoding a phosphate transferase (Acp) involved in the maintenance of the acetyl phosphate pool in the cell [405]. Ribosomal synthesis (ribosomal release factor and 50S ribosomal protein L7/L12), proteins involved in the energy pathway (Succinyl-CoA synthetase α and β chains) and proteins that could contribute to synthesis of the efflux system (possible membrane fusion component of efflux system, putative ABC transport system ATP-binding protein) were also upregulated in both immobilized cells and biofilms of *C. jejuni* [179, 335]. This would indicate that the biofilm formation comes with induced systems that would protect the cells against adverse conditions. However, it is not known whether those systems are induced by the nutrient depletion in the spent medium, which could initiate the biofilm formation or whether the specific biofilm environment is responsible for the induction of these regulations. It is possible that the biological responses of the biofilm structure could be induced by specific environmental threats or only one specific threat could be responsible for the regulation of a set of biological defences.

In conclusion, *Campylobacter* has the ability to be organized into a biofilm structure through a net of exopolymeric substances connected to the cells or the microcolonies. It is able to attach to various inert surfaces and to form different types of biofilm. No mode of growth has been yet described concerning the development of *Campylobacter* on biological surfaces. The window of growth of *Campylobacter* is narrow considering the range of temperatures, pH and oxygen concentrations. However, this pathogen is frequently detected in environments out of the range of its growth conditions. Considering the idiosyncrasy of *Campylobacter*, the biofilm could be a protective structure that could insure the survival of this pathogen during the transition towards favourable growth environments such as the intestinal tract of birds or mammalian organisms.

Chapter VI

General Conclusion

Before colonisation of human intestinal tract, *C. jejuni* has to cope with environmental stresses: starvation, aerobic environments, low temperatures, low pH and exposition to antibiotics. In spite of its apparent sensitivity (microaerophilic and thermophilic characteristics), *C. jejuni* still represents a conundrum for public health authorities, as it is responsible for most of the bacterial human gastro-enteritis throughout the world. Several *C. jejuni* genome sequences are now completely available and additionnal sequencing projects are in process of assemblage. Analysis of these data already gives new insights on the particularities of this pathogen. Like *H. pylori*, *C. jejuni* possesses only three predicted σ factors (rpoD, rpoN, fliA). Many key regulators of the stress defence response are absent from its genome even if 28 % of *C. jejuni* genes show closest similarity to *E. coli* and 27 % to *B. subtilis*. Interestingly, as for the oxydative and thermal stress responses *C. jejuni* seems to use sophisticated combined regulation mechanisms alternatively closest to *E. coli* or *B. subtilis* paradigms. Despite the genomic data, many adaptative responses (cold shock, starvation, low pH resistance) of this bacterium are still unknown or poorly understood. *C. jejuni* is thought to adopt a viable but non culturable (VBNC) form in unfavourable conditions. These forms conserve a metabolic activity and are able to recover a cultivable and fully virulent state when replaced in favourable conditions. It is not clear whether this particular state is a degenerative form or a survival strategy, but it is often described as playing a role in resistance to cold temperature, starvation, osmotic changes and oxidative stress.

In the current chapter, a special emphasis has been done on the alternative strategies of *Campylobacter* to adapt to the environment. *Campylobacter* membranes as the centrepiece of sensing and adaptative response system have been highlighted. Special capacities such as antibioresistance, chemiotaxis, motility or biofilm formation have been reviewed to explore their role in the *Campylobacter* adaptation in the environment. All these combined data demonstrate in spite of its small genome, its lack in regulatory systems and its relative sensitivity, *C. jejuni* possesses a set of adapted responses to survive severe stresses. As it represents a major microbiological risk, adapted measures have to be taken from broiler stocks to kitchens in order to reduce its impact on public health.

References

[1] Acik, M.N. and Cetinkaya, B. (2005) The heterogeneity of *Campylobacter jejuni* and *Campylobacter coli* strains isolated from healthy cattle. *Lett. Appl. Microbiol,* 41, 397-403.

[2] Acke, E., Whyte, P., Jones, B.R., McGill, K., Collins, J.D. and Fanning, S. (2006) Prevalence of thermophilic *Campylobacter* species in cats and dogs in two animal shelters in Ireland. *Vet. Rec,* 158, 51-54.

[3] Adak, G.K., Cowden, J.M., Nicholas, S. and Evans, H.S. (1995) The Public Health Laboratory Service national case-control study of primary indigenous sporadic cases of campylobacter infection. *Epidemiol. Infect,* 115, 15-22.

[4] Adhikari, B., Connolly, J.H., Madie, P. and Davies, P.R. (2004) Prevalence and clonal diversity of *Campylobacter* jejuni from dairy farms and urban sources. *N. Z. Vet. J,* 52, 378-383.

[5] Adkin, A., Hartnett, E., Jordan, L., Newell, D. and Davison, H. (2006) Use of a systematic review to assist the development of *Campylobacter* control strategies in broilers. *J. Appl. Microbiol,* 100, 306-315.

[6] Akiba, M., Lin, J., Barton, Y.W. and Zhang, Q. (2006) Interaction of CmeABC and CmeDEF in conferring antimicrobial resistance and maintaining cell viability in *Campylobacter jejuni*. *J. Antimicrob. Chemother,* 57, 52-60.

[7] Alamuri, P. and Maier, R.J. (2006) Methionine sulfoxide reductase in *Helicobacter pylori:* interaction with methionine-rich proteins and stress-induced expression. *J. Bacteriol,* 188, 5839-5850.

[8] Alfredson, D.A. and Korolik, V. (2003) Sequence analysis of a cryptic plasmid pCJ419 from *Campylobacter jejuni* and construction of an *Escherichia coli-Campylobacter* shuttle vector. *Plasmid*, 50, 152-160.

[9] Allos, B.M. (2001) *Campylobacter jejuni* Infections: update on emerging issues and trends. *Clin. Infect. Dis,* 32, 1201-1206.

[10] Alter, T., Gaull, F., Kasimir, S., Gurtler, M., Mielke, H., Linnebur, M. and Fehlhaber, K. (2005) Prevalences and transmission routes of *Campylobacter* spp. strains within multiple pig farms. *Vet. Microbiol,* 108, 251-261.

[11] Alter, T. and Scherer, K. (2006) Stress response of *Campylobacter* spp. and its role in food processing. *J. Vet. Med. [B],* 53, 351-357.

[12] Amici, A., Levine, R.L., Tsai, L. and Stadtman, E.R. (1989) Conversion of amino acid residues in proteins and amino acid homopolymers to carbonyl derivatives by metal-catalyzed oxidation reactions. *J. Biol. Chem,* 264, 3341-3346.

[13] Andersen, M.T., Brondsted, L., Pearson, B.M., Mulholland, F., Parker, M., Pin, C., Wells, J.M. and Ingmer, H. (2005) Diverse roles for HspR in *Campylobacter jejuni* revealed by the proteome, transcriptome and phenotypic characterization of an hspR mutant. *Microbiology,* 151, 905-915.

[14] Annual Report 2005 on Zoonoses in Denmark [online] The Ministry of Family and Consumer Affairs (2006) Copenhagen, Denmark, Available from: http://www.food.dtu.dk/Admin/Public/DWSDownload.aspx?File=Files%2fFiler%2fZoonosecentret%2fPublikationer%2fAnnual+Report%2fAnnual_Report_2005_med_farvebilleder.pdf.

[15] Armitage, J.P. (1999) Bacterial tactic responses. *Adv. Microb. Physiol,* 41, 229-289.

[16] Arora, S.K., Ritchings, B.W., Almira, E.C., Lory, S. and Ramphal, R. (1997) A transcriptional activator, FleQ, regulates mucin adhesion and flagellar gene expression in *Pseudomonas aeruginosa* in a cascade manner. *J. Bacteriol,* 179, 5574-5581.

[17] Aspinall, G.O., McDonald, A.G., Raju, T.S., Pang, H., Moran, A.P. and Penner, J.L. (1993) Chemical structures of the core regions of *Campylobacter jejuni* serotypes O:1, O:4, O:23, and O:36 lipopolysaccharides. *Eur. J. Biochem,* 213, 1017-1027.

[18] Aspinall, G.O., Lynch, C.M., Pang, H., Shaver, R.T. and Moran, A.P. (1995) Chemical structures of the core region of *Campylobacter jejuni* O:3 lipopolysaccharide and an associated polysaccharide. *Eur. J. Biochem,* 231, 570-578.

[19] Avrain, L., Allain, L., Vernozy-Rozand, C. and Kempf, I. (2003) Disinfectant susceptibility testing of avian and swine *Campylobacter* isolates by a filtration method. *Vet. Microbiol,* 96, 35-40.

[20] Bachoual, R., Ouabdesselam, S., Mory, F., Lascols, C., Soussy, C.J. and Tankovic, J. (2001) Single or double mutational alterations of *gyrA* associated with fluoroquinolone resistance in *Campylobacter jejuni* and *Campylobacter coli. Microb. Drug Resist,* 7, 257-261.

[21] Bacon, D.J., Alm, R.A., Hu, L., Hickey, T.E., Ewing, C.P., Batchelor, R.A., Trust, T.J. and Guerry, P. (2002) DNA sequence and mutational analyses of the pVir plasmid of *Campylobacter jejuni* 81-176. *Infect Immun,* 70, 6242-6250.

[22] Baffone, W., Casaroli, A., Citterio, B., Pierfelici, L., Campana, R., Vittoria, E., Guaglianone, E. and Donelli, G. (2006) *Campylobacter jejuni* loss of culturability in aqueous microcosms and ability to resuscitate in a mouse model. *Int J Food Microbiol,* 107, 83-91.

[23] Bailey, G.D., Vanselow, B.A., Hornitzky, M.A., Hum, S.I., Eamens, G.J., Gill, P.A., Walker, K.H. and Cronin, J.P. (2003) A study of the foodborne pathogens: *Campylobacter, Listeria* and *Yersinia,* in faeces from slaughter-age cattle and sheep in Australia. *Commun Dis Intell,* 27, 249-257.

[24] Baillon, M.L., van Vliet, A.H., Ketley, J.M., Constantinidou, C. and Penn, C.W. (1999) An iron-regulated alkyl hydroperoxide reductase (AhpC) confers aerotolerance and oxidative stress resistance to the microaerophilic pathogen *Campylobacter jejuni. J Bacteriol,* 181, 4798-4804.

[25] Barnard, F.M., Loughlin, M.F., Fainberg, H.P., Messenger, M.P., Ussery, D.W., Williams, P. and Jenks, P.J. (2004) Global regulation of virulence and the stress response by CsrA in the highly adapted human gastric pathogen *Helicobacter pylori. Mol. Microbiol,* 51, 15-32.

[26] Bashor, M.P., Curtis, P.A., Keener, K.M., Sheldon, B.W., Kathariou, S. and Osborne, J.A. (2004) Effects of carcass washers on *Campylobacter* contamination in large broiler processing plants. *Poult. Sci,* 83, 1232-1239.

[27] Basu, M., Czinn, S.J. and Blanchard, T.G. (2004) Absence of catalase reduces long-term survival of *Helicobacter pylori* in macrophage phagosomes. *Helicobacter,* 9, 211-216.
[28] Batchelor, R.A., Pearson, B.M., Friis, L.M., Guerry, P. and Wells, J.M. (2004) Nucleotide sequences and comparison of two large conjugative plasmids from different *Campylobacter* species. *Microbiology,* 150, 3507-3517.
[29] Bender, J.B., Shulman, S.A., Averbeck, G.A., Pantlin, G.C. and Stromberg, B.E. (2005) Epidemiologic features of *Campylobacter* infection among cats in the upper midwestern United States. *J. Am. Vet. Med. Assoc,* 226, 544-547.
[30] Berlett, B.S. and Stadtman, E.R. (1997) Protein oxidation in aging, disease, and oxidative stress. *J. Biol. Chem,* 272, 20313-20316.
[31] Besser, T.E., Lejeune, J.T., Rice, D.H., Berg, J., Stilborn, R.P., Kaya, K., Bae, W. and Hancock, D.D. (2005) Increasing prevalence of *Campylobacter jejuni* in feedlot cattle through the feeding period. *Appl. Environ. Microbiol,* 71, 5752-5758.
[32] Beumer, R.R., Noomen, A., Marijs, J.A. and Kampelmacher, E. (1985) Antibacterial action of the lactoperoxidase on *Campylobacter jejuni* in cow's milk. *Nether Milk Dairy J,* 39, 107-114.
[33] Bhaduri, S. and Cottrell, B. (2004) Survival of cold-stressed *Campylobacter jejuni* on ground chicken and chicken skin during frozen storage. *Appl. Environ. Microbiol,* 70, 7103-7109.
[34] Black, R.E., Levine, M.M., Clements, M.L., Hughes, T.P. and Blaser, M.J. (1988) Experimental *Campylobacter jejuni* infection in humans. *J. Infect. Dis,* 157, 472-479.
[35] Bladergroen, M.R., Badelt, K. and Spaink, H.P. (2003) Infection-blocking genes of a symbiotic *Rhizobium leguminosarum* strain that are involved in temperature-dependent protein secretion. *Mol. Plant-Microbe Interact,* 16, 53-64.
[36] Blaser, M.J., Hardesty, H.L., Powers, B. and Wang, W.L.L. (1980) Survival of *Campylobacter fetus* subsp. *jejuni* in biological milieus. *J. Clin. Microbiol,* 11, 309-313.
[37] Bohin, J.-P. (2000) Osmoregulated periplasmic glucans in Proteobacteria. *FEMS Microbiol. Lett,* 186, 11-19.
[38] Bol, D.K. and Yasbin, R.E. (1990) Characterization of an inducible oxidative stress system in *Bacillus subtilis*. *J. Bacteriol,* 172, 3503-3506.

[39] Bolla, J.M., Loret, E., Zalewski, M. and Pages, J.M. (1995) Conformational analysis of the *Campylobacter jejuni* porin. *J. Bacteriol*, 177, 4266-4271.

[40] Bolla, J.M., De, E., Dorez, A. and Pages, J.M. (2000) Purification, characterization and sequence analysis of Omp50, a new porin isolated from *Campylobacter jejuni*. *Biochem. J*, 352, 637-643.

[41] Bolton, F.J., Wareing, D.R.A., Skirrow, M.B. and Hutchinson, D.N. (1992) Identification and biotyping of campylobacters. In: R.G. Board, D. Jones and F.A. Skinner (Eds.). *Identification methods in applied and environmental microbiology*. London: Blackwell Scientific; 151-161.

[42] Botsford, J.L. and Drexler, M. (1978) The cyclic 3',5'-adenosine monophosphate receptor protein and regulation of cyclic 3',5'-adenosine monophosphate synthesis in *Escherichia coli*. *Mol. Gen. Genet*, 165, 47-56.

[43] Bovill, R.A. and Mackey, B.M. (1997) Resuscitation of 'non-culturable' cells from aged cultures of *Campylobacter jejuni*. *Microbiology*, 143 (Pt 5), 1575-1581.

[44] Boyd, Y., Herbert, E.G., Marston, K.L., Jones, M.A. and Barrow, P.A. (2005) Host genes affect intestinal colonisation of newly hatched chickens by *Campylobacter jejuni*. *Immunogenetics*, 57, 248-253.

[45] Boysen, L., Knochel, S. and Rosenquist, H. (2007) Survival of *Campylobacter jejuni* in different gas mixtures. *FEMS Microbiol. Lett*, 266, 152-157.

[46] Bras, A.M., Chatterjee, S., Wren, B.W., Newell, D.G. and Ketley, J.M. (1999) A novel *Campylobacter jejuni* two-component regulatory system important for temperature-dependent growth and colonization. *J. Bacteriol*, 181, 3298-3302.

[47] Briolat, V. and Reysset, G. (2002) Identification of the *Clostridium perfringens* genes involved in the adaptive response to oxidative stress. *J. Bacteriol*, 184, 2333-2343.

[48] Brondsted, L., Andersen, M.T., Parker, M., Jorgensen, K. and Ingmer, H. (2005) The HtrA protease of *Campylobacter jejuni* is required for heat and oxygen tolerance and for optimal interaction with human epithelial cells. *Appl. Environ. Microbiol*, 71, 3205-3212.

[49] Brown, J.L., Ross, T., McMeekin, T.A. and Nichols, P.D. (1997) Acid habituation of *Escherichia coli* and the potential role of cyclopropane fatty acids in low pH tolerance. *Int. J. Food Microbiol*, 37, 163-173.

[50] Bsat, N., Herbig, A., Casillas-Martinez, L., Setlow, P. and Helmann, J.D. (1998) *Bacillus subtilis* contains multiple Fur homologues: identification of the iron uptake (Fur) and peroxide regulon (PerR) repressors. *Mol. Microbiol,* 29, 189-198.

[51] Bull, S.A., Allen, V.M., Domingue, G., Jorgensen, F., Frost, J.A., Ure, R., Whyte, R., Tinker, D., Corry, J.E., Gillard-King, J. and Humphrey, T.J. (2006) Sources of *Campylobacter* spp. colonizing housed broiler flocks during rearing. *Appl. Environ. Microbiol,* 72, 645-652.

[52] Bury-Mone, S., Kaakoush, N.O., Asencio, C., Megraud, F., Thibonnier, M., De Reuse, H. and Mendz, G.L. (2006) Is *Helicobacter pylori* a true microaerophile? *Helicobacter,* 11, 296-303.

[53] Buswell, C.M., Herlihy, Y.M., Lawrence, L.M., McGuiggan, J.T.M., Marsh, P.D., Keevil, C.W. and Leach, S.A. (1998) Extended survival and persistence of *Campylobacter* spp. in water and aquatic biofilms and their detection by immunofluorescent-antibody and -rRNA staining. *Appl. Environ. Microbiol,* 64, 733-741.

[54] Butler, R.C., Lund, V. and Carlson, D.A. (1987) Susceptibility of *Campylobacter jejuni* and *Yersinia enterocolitica* to UV radiation. *Appl. Environ. Microbiol,* 53, 375-378.

[55] Bywater, R.J. (2004) Veterinary use of antimicrobials and emergence of resistance in zoonotic and sentinel bacteria in the EU. *J. Vet. Med.* [B], 51, 361-363.

[56] Cagliero, C., Mouline, C., Payot, S. and Cloeckaert, A. (2005) Involvement of the CmeABC efflux pump in the macrolide resistance of *Campylobacter coli. J. Antimicrob. Chemother,* 56, 948-950.

[57] Cagliero, C., Maurel, M.C., Cloeckaert, A. and Payot, S. (2007) Regulation of the expression of the CmeABC efflux pump in *Campylobacter jejuni*: identification of a point mutation abolishing the binding of the CmeR repressor in an in vitro-selected multidrug-resistant mutant. *FEMS Microbiol. Lett,* 267, 89-94.

[58] Calamita, G., Bishai, W.R., Preston, G.M., Guggino, W.B. and Agre, P. (1995) Molecular cloning and characterization of AqpZ, a water channel from *Escherichia coli. J. Biol. Chem,* 270, 29063-29066.

[59] Caldwell, M.B., Guerry, P., Lee, E.C., Burans, J.P. and Walker, R.I. (1985) Reversible expression of flagella in *Campylobacter jejuni. Infect. Immun,* 50, 941-943.

[60] Cappelier, J.M., Lazaro, B., Rossero, A., Fernandez-Astorga, A. and Federighi, M. (1997) Double staining (CTC-DAPI) for detection and enumeration of viable but non-culturable *Campylobacter jejuni* cells. *Vet. Res,* 28, 547-555.

[61] Cappelier, J.M., Rossero, A. and Federighi, M. (2000) Demonstration of a protein synthesis in starved *Campylobacter jejuni* cells. *Int. J. Food Microbiol,* 55, 63-67.

[62] Carlsson, J. and Carpenter, V.S. (1980) The recA+ gene product is more important than catalase and superoxide dismutase in protecting *Escherichia coli* against hydrogen peroxide toxicity. *J. Bacteriol,* 142, 319-321.

[63] Carrillo, C.D., Taboada, E., Nash, J.H.E., Lanthier, P., Kelly, J., Lau, P.C., Verhulp, R., Mykytczuk, O., Sy, J., Findlay, W.A., Amoako, K., Gomis, S., Willson, P., Austin, J.W., Potter, A., Babiuk, L., Allan, B. and Szymanski, C.M. (2004) Genome-wide Expression Analyses of *Campylobacter jejuni* NCTC11168 Reveals Coordinate Regulation of Motility and Virulence by flhA. *J. Biol. Chem,* 279, 20327-20338.

[64] Cashel, M., Gentry, D.M., Hernandez, V.J. and Vinella, D. (1996) The stringent response. In: F.C. Neidhardt, R. Curtiss, J.L. Ingraham, E.C.C. Lin, K.B. Low, B. Magasanik, W.S. Reznikoff, M. Riley, M. Schaechter and H.E. Umbarger (Eds.). *Escherichia coli* and *Salmonella typhimurium*: Cellular and Molecular Biology. Washington D.C.: American Society for Microbiology; 1458-1496.

[65] Casillas-Martinez, L. and Setlow, P. (1997) Alkyl hydroperoxide reductase, catalase, MrgA, and superoxide dismutase are not involved in resistance of *Bacillus subtilis* spores to heat or oxidizing agents. *J. Bacteriol,* 179, 7420-7425.

[66] Cawthraw, S., Ayling, R., Nuijten, P., Wassenaar, T. and Newell, D.G. (1994) Isotype, specificity, and kinetics of systemic and mucosal antibodies to Campylobacter jejuni antigens, including flagellin, during experimental oral infections of chickens. *Avian Dis,* 38, 341-349.

[67] Chang, Y.Y. and Cronan, J.E., Jr. (1999) Membrane cyclopropane fatty acid content is a major factor in acid resistance of *Escherichia coli. Mol. Microbiol,* 33, 249-259.

[68] Characklis, W.G. and Marshall, K.C. (1990) Biofilms: a basis for an interdisciplinary approach. In: W.G. Characklis and K.C. Marshall (Eds.). *Biofilms.* New York: Wiley; 3-15.

[69] Chaveerach, P., Keuzenkamp, D.A., Urlings, H.A.P., Lipman, L.J.A. and van Knapen, F. (2001) In vitro study on the effect of organic acids on *Campylobacter jejuni/coli* populations in mixtures of water and feed. *Poult. Sci,* 81, 621-628.

[70] Chaveerach, P., ter Huurne, A.A., Lipman, L.J. and van Knapen, F. (2003) Survival and resuscitation of ten strains of *Campylobacter jejuni* and *Campylobacter coli* under acid conditions. *Appl. Environ. Microbiol,* 69, 711-714.

[71] Chevalier, C., Thiberge, J.M., Ferrero, R.L. and Labigne, A. (1999) Essential role of *Helicobacter pylori* gamma-glutamyltranspeptidase for the colonization of the gastric mucosa of mice. *Mol. Microbiol,* 31, 1359-1372.

[72] Choi, H.K., Marth, E.H. and Vasadava, P.C. (1993) Use of microwave to inactivate *Yersinia enterocolitica* and *Campylobacter jejuni* in milk. *Milchwissenschaft,* 48, 134-136.

[73] Choi, S.H., Baumler, D.J. and Kaspar, C.W. (2000) Contribution of dps to acid stress tolerance and oxidative stress tolerance in *Escherichia coli* O157:H7. *Appl. Environ. Microbiol,* 66, 3911-3916.

[74] Christopher, F.M., Smith, G.C. and Vanderzant, C. (1982) Examination of poultry giblets, raw milk and meat for *Campylobacter fetus* subsp. *jejuni*. *J. Food Prot,* 45, 260-262.

[75] Coloe, P.J., Slattery, J.F., Cavanaugh, P. and Vaughan, J. (1986) The cellular fatty acid composition of *Campylobacter* species isolated from cases of enteritis in man and animals. *J. Hyg.* (Lond.), 96, 225-229.

[76] Corcoran, D., Quinn, T., Cotter, L., O'Halloran, F. and Fanning, S. (2005) Characterisation of a *cmeABC* operon in a quinolone-resistant *Campylobacter coli* isolate of Irish origin. *Microb. Drug Resist,* 11, 303-308.

[77] Costerton, J.W., Lewandowski, Z., Caldwell, D.E., Korber, D.R. and Lappin-Scott, H.M. (1995) Microbial Biofilms. *Annu. Rev. Microbiol,* 49, 711-745.

[78] Cronan, J.E., Jr. (1968) Phospholipid alterations during growth of *Escherichia coli. J. Bacteriol,* 95, 2054-2061.

[79] Cronan, J.E., Jr., Nunn, W.D. and Batchelor, J.G. (1974) Studies on the biosynthesis of cyclopropane fatty acids in *Escherichia coli. Biochim. Biophys. Acta,* 348, 63-75.

[80] Cuk, Z., Annan-Prah, A., Janc, M. and Zajc-Satler, J. (1987) Yoghurt: an unlikely source of *Campylobacter jejuni/coli*. *J. Appl. Bacteriol,* 63, 201-5.

[81] Day, W.A., Jr., Sajecki, J.L., Pitts, T.M. and Joens, L.A. (2000) Role of catalase in *Campylobacter jejuni* intracellular survival. *Infect. Immun,* 68, 6337-6345.

[82] De, E., Jullien, M., Labesse, G., Pages, J.M., Molle, G. and Bolla, J.M. (2000) MOMP (major outer membrane protein) of *Campylobacter jejuni*; a versatile pore-forming protein. *FEBS Lett,* 469, 93-97.

[83] de Jonge, R., Ritmeester, W.S. and van Leusden, F.M. (2003) Adaptive responses of *Salmonella enterica* serovar Typhimurium DT104 and other *S.* Typhimurium strains and *Escherichia coli* O157 to low pH environments. *J. Appl. Microbiol,* 94, 625-632.

[84] de Zoete, M.R., van Putten, J.P. and Wagenaar, J.A. (2006) Vaccination of chickens against *Campylobacter*. Vaccine, *in press*.

[85] Dedieu, L., Pages, J.M. and Bolla, J.M. (2002) Environmental regulation of *Campylobacter jejuni* major outer membrane protein porin expression in *Escherichia coli* monitored by using green fluorescent protein. *Appl. Environ. Microbiol,* 68, 4209-4215.

[86] Dedieu, L., Pages, J.M. and Bolla, J.M. (2004) Use of the *omp50* gene for identification of *Campylobacter* species by PCR. *J. Clin. Microbiol,* 42, 2301-2305.

[87] Deming, M.S., Tauxe, R.V., Blake, P.A., Dixon, S.E., Fowler, B.S., Jones, T.S., Lockamy, E.A., Patton, C.M. and Sikes, R.O. (1987) *Campylobacter* enteritis at a university: transmission from eating chicken and from cats. *Am. J. Epidemiol,* 126, 526-534.

[88] Denich, T.J., Beaudette, L.A., Lee, H. and Trevors, J.T. (2003) Effect of selected environmental and physico-chemical factors on bacterial cytoplasmic membranes. *J. Microbiol. Meth,* 52, 149-182.

[89] Desnues, B., Cuny, C., Gregori, G., Dukan, S., Aguilaniu, H. and Nystrom, T. (2003) Differential oxidative damage and expression of stress defence regulons in culturable and non-culturable *Escherichia coli* cells. *EMBO Rep,* 4, 400-404.

[90] Diker, K.S., Akan, M., Hascelik, G. and Yurdakok, M. (1991) The bactericidal activity of tea against *Campylobacter jejuni* and *Campylobacter coli*. *Lett. Appl. Microbiol,* 12, 34-35.

[91] Dingle, K.E., Colles, F.M., Wareing, D.R., Ure, R., Fox, A.J., Bolton, F.E., Bootsma, H.J., Willems, R.J., Urwin, R. and Maiden, M.C. (2001) Multilocus sequence typing system for *Campylobacter jejuni*. *J. Clin. Microbiol,* 39, 14-23.

[92] Dingle, K.E., Colles, F.M., Ure, R., Wagenaar, J.A., Duim, B., Bolton, F.J., Fox, A.J., Wareing, D.R. and Maiden, M.C. (2002) Molecular characterization of *Campylobacter jejuni* clones: a basis for epidemiologic investigation. *Emerg. Infect. Dis,* 8, 949-55.

[93] Doerrler, W.T. (2006) Lipid trafficking to the outer membrane of Gram-negative bacteria. *Mol Microbiol,* 60, 542-552.

[94] Dorrell, N., Mangan, J.A., Laing, K.G., Hinds, J., Linton, D., Al-Ghusein, H., Barrell, B.G., Parkhill, J., Stoker, N.G., Karlyshev, A.V., Butcher, P.D. and Wren, B.W. (2001) Whole genome comparison of *Campylobacter jejuni* human isolates using a low-cost microarray reveals extensive genetic diversity. *Genome Res,* 11, 1706-1715.

[95] Doyle, M.P. and Erickson, M.C. (2006) Reducing the carriage of foodborne pathogens in livestock and poultry. *Poult. Sci,* 85, 960-973.

[96] Driks, A. (2007) Surface appendages of bacterial spores. Mol Microbiol, 63, 623-625.

[97] Duffy, L. and Dykes, G.A. (2006) Growth temperature of four *Campylobacter jejuni* strains influences their subsequent survival in food and water. *Lett. Appl. Microbiol,* 43, 596-601.

[98] Dykes, G.A. and Moorhead, S.M. (2001) Survival of *Campylobacter jejuni* on vacuum or carbon dioxide packaged primal beef cuts stored à -1.5°C. *Food Control,* 12, 553-557.

[99] Dykes, G.A., Sampathkumar, B. and Korber, D.R. (2003) Planktonic or biofilm growth affects survival, hydrophobicity and protein expression patterns of a pathogenic *Campylobacter jejuni* strain. *Int. J. Food Microbiol,* 89, 1-10.

[100] Eberhart-Phillips, J., Walker, N., Garrett, N., Bell, D., Sinclair, D., Rainger, W. and Bates, M. (1997) Campylobacteriosis in New Zealand: results of a case-control study. *J. Epidemiol. Commun Health,* 51, 686-91.

[101] Effler, P., Leong, M.C., Kimura, A., Nakata, M., Burr, R., Cremer, E. and Slutsker, L. (2001) Sporadic *Campylobacter jejuni* in Hawaï : association with prior antibiotic use and commercially prepared chicken. *J. Infect,* 183, 1152-1155.

[102] Elvers, K.T., Turner, S.M., Wainwright, L.M., Marsden, G., Hinds, J., Cole, J.A., Poole, R.K., Penn, C.W. and Park, S.F. (2005) NssR, a member of the Crp-Fnr superfamily from *Campylobacter jejuni*, regulates a nitrosative stress-responsive regulon that includes both a single-domain and a truncated haemoglobin. *Mol. Microbiol*, 57, 735-750.

[103] Engelmann, S. and Hecker, M. (1996) Impaired oxidative stress resistance of *Bacillus subtilis* sigB mutants and the role of katA and katE. *FEMS Microbiol. Lett*, 145, 63-69.

[104] Fabret, C., Feher, V.A. and Hoch, J.A. (1999) Two-Component Signal Transduction in *Bacillus subtilis*: How One Organism Sees Its World. *J. Bacteriol*, 181, 1975-1983.

[105] Farber, J.M. and Levine, R.L. (1986) Sequence of a peptide susceptible to mixed-function oxidation. Probable cation binding site in glutamine synthetase. *J. Biol. Chem*, 261, 4574-4578.

[106] Farr, S.B. and Kogoma, T. (1991) Oxidative stress responses in *Escherichia coli* and *Salmonella typhimurium*. *Microbiol. Rev.*, 55, 561-585.

[107] Farrell, M.J. and Finkel, S.E. (2003) The growth advantage in stationary-phase phenotype conferred by rpoS mutations is dependent on the pH and nutrient environment. *J. Bacteriol*, 185, 7044-7052.

[108] Federighi, M., Cappelier, J.M., Rossero, A., Coppen, P. and Denis, J.C. (1995) Assessment of the effect of a treatment of whole chicken carcasses on *Campylobacter* spp. *Sci. Alim.*, 15, 393-401.

[109] Federighi, M., Tholozan, J.L., Cappelier, J.M., Tissier, J.P. and Jouve, J.L. (1998) Evidence of non-coccoid viable but non-culturable *Campylobacter jejuni* cells in microcosm water by direct viable count, CTC-DAPI double staining, and scanning electron microscopy. *Food Microbiol*, 15, 539-550.

[110] Federighi, M. (1999) *Campylobacter* et Hygiène des Aliments. Paris: Economica.

[111] Fisher, K. and Phillips, C.A. (2006) The effect of lemon, orange and bergamot essential oils and their components on the survival of *Campylobacter jejuni, Escherichia coli* O157, *Listeria monocytogenes, Bacillus cereus* and *Staphylococcus aureus* in vitro and in food systems. *J. Appl. Microbiol*, 101, 1232-1240.

[112] Fisher, M.T. and Stadtman, E.R. (1992) Oxidative modification of *Escherichia coli* glutamine synthetase. Decreases in the thermodynamic stability of protein structure and specific changes in the active site conformation. *J. Biol. Chem,* 267, 1872-1880.

[113] Fouts, D.E., Mongodin, E.F., Mandrell, R.E., Miller, W.G., Rasko, D.A., Ravel, J., Brinkac, L.M., DeBoy, R.T., Parker, C.T., Daugherty, S.C., Dodson, R.J., Durkin, A.S., Madupu, R., Sullivan, S.A., Shetty, J.U., Ayodeji, M.A., Shvartsbeyn, A., Schatz, M.C., Badger, J.H., Fraser, C.M. and Nelson, K.E. (2005) Major structural differences and novel potential virulence mechanisms from the genomes of multiple *Campylobacter* species. *PLoS Biol,* 3, e15.

[114] French, N., Barrigas, M., Brown, P., Ribiero, P., Williams, N., Leatherbarrow, H., Birtles, R., Bolton, E., Fearnhead, P. and Fox, A. (2005) Spatial epidemiology and natural population structure of *Campylobacter jejuni* colonizing a farmland ecosystem. *Environ. Microbiol,* 7, 1116-1126.

[115] Fridovich, I. (1989) Superoxide dismutases. An adaptation to a paramagnetic gas. *J. Biol. Chem,* 264, 7761-7764.

[116] Fridovich, I. (1998) Oxygen toxicity: a radical explanation. *J Exp Biol,* 201, 1203-1209.

[117] Friedman, C.R., Neimann, J., Wegener, H.C. and Tauxe, R.V. (2000) Epidemiology of *Campylobacter jejuni* infections in the United States and other industrialized nations. In: I. Nachamkin and M.J. Blaser (Eds.). Campylobacter. Washington D.C.: ASM Press; 121-138.

[118] Friedman, C.R., Hoekstra, R.M., Samuel, M., Marcus, R., Bender, J., Shiferaw, B., Reddy, S., Ahuja, S.D., Helfrick, D.L., Hardnett, F., Carter, M., Anderson, B. and Tauxe, R.V. (2004) Risk factors for sporadic *Campylobacter* infection in the United States: A case-control study in FoodNet sites. *Clin. Infect. Dis,* 38 Suppl 3, S285-S296.

[119] Fry, B.N., Feng, S., Chen, Y.Y., Newell, D.G., Coloe, P.J. and Korolik, V. (2000) The galE gene of *Campylobacter jejuni* is involved in lipopolysaccharide synthesis and virulence. *Infect. Immun,* 68, 2594-2601.

[120] Fuangthong, M., Herbig, A.F., Bsat, N. and Helmann, J.D. (2002) Regulation of the *Bacillus subtilis* fur and perR genes by PerR: not all members of the PerR regulon are peroxide inducible. *J. Bacteriol,* 184, 3276-3286.

[121] Fullerton, K.E., Ingram, L.A., Jones, T.F., Anderson, B.J., McCarthy, P.V., Hurd, S., Shiferaw, B., Vugia, D., Haubert, N., Hayes, T., Wedel, S., Scallan, E., Henao, O. and Angulo, F.J. (2007) Sporadic *Campylobacter* infection in infants: a population-based surveillance case-control study. *Pediatr. Infect. Dis. J*, 26, 19-24.

[122] Galinski, E.A. (1995) Osmoadaptation in bacteria. Adv Microb Physiol, 37, 272-328.

[123] Gate, L., Paul, J., Ba, G.N., Tew, K.D. and Tapiero, H. (1999) Oxidative stress induced in pathologies: the role of antioxidants. *Biomed. Pharmacother*, 53, 169-180.

[124] Gaynor, E.C., Wells, D.H., MacKichan, J.K. and Falkow, S. (2005) The *Campylobacter jejuni* stringent response controls specific stress survival and virulence-associated phenotypes. *Mol. Microbiol*, 56, 8-27.

[125] Ge, B., McDermott, G., White, D.G. and Meng, J. (2005) Role of efflux pumps and topoisomerase mutations in fluoroquinolone resistance in *Campylobacter jejuni* and *Campylobacter coli*. *Antimicrob. Agents Chemother*, 49, 3347-3354.

[126] Gorden, J. and Small, P.L. (1993) Acid resistance in enteric bacteria. *Infect. Immun*, 61, 364-367.

[127] Gosink, K.K., Buron-Barral, M.C. and Parkinson, J.S. (2006) Signaling interactions between the aerotaxis transducer Aer and heterologous chemoreceptors in *Escherichia coli*. *J. Bacteriol*, 188, 3487-3493.

[128] Goswami, M., Mangoli, S.H. and Jawali, N. (2006) Involvement of reactive oxygen species in the action of ciprofloxacin against *Escherichia coli*. *Antimicrob. Agents Chemother*, 50, 949-954.

[129] Gouffi, K. and Blanco, C. (2000) Is the accumulation of osmoprotectant the unique mechanism involved in bacterial osmoprotection? *Int. J. Food Microbiol*, 55, 171-174.

[130] Grajewski, B.A., Kusek, J.W. and Gelfand, H.M. (1985) Development of a bacteriophage typing system for *Campylobacter jejuni* and *Campylobacter coli*. *J. Clin. Microbiol*, 22, 13-18.

[131] Grinberg, A., Pomroy, W.E., Weston, J.F., Ayanegui-Alcerreca, A. and Knight, D. (2005) The occurrence of *Cryptosporidium parvum, Campylobacter* and *Salmonella* in newborn dairy calves in the Manawatu region of New Zealand. *N. Z. Vet. J*, 53, 315-320.

[132] Grogan, D.W. and Cronan, J.E., Jr. (1986) Characterization of *Escherichia coli* mutants completely defective in synthesis of cyclopropane fatty acids. *J. Bacteriol*, 166, 872-877.

[133] Grogan, D.W. and Cronan, J.E., Jr. (1997) Cyclopropane ring formation in membrane lipids of bacteria. *Microbiol. Mol. Biol. Rev,* 61, 429-441.
[134] Guckert, J.B., Hood, M.A. and White, D.C. (1986) Phospholipid ester-linked fatty acid profile changes during nutrient deprivation of *Vibrio cholerae*: increases in the trans/cis ratio and proportions of cyclopropyl fatty acids. *Appl. Environ. Microbiol,* 52, 794-801.
[135] Guerra, D.J. and Browse, J.A. (1990) *Escherichia coli* beta-hydroxydecanoyl thioester dehydrase reacts with native C10 acyl-acyl-carrier proteins of plant and bacterial origin. *Arch. Biochem. Biophys,* 280, 336-345.
[136] Guerry, P., Alm, R.A., Power, M.E., Logan, S.M. and Trust, T.J. (1991) Role of two flagellin genes in *Campylobacter* motility. *J. Bacteriol,* 173, 4757-4764.
[137] Gundogdu, O. Updated (2006) *Campylobacter jejuni* NCTC11168 genome [online]. [Last accessed on 25/01/2007]. Available from: http://www.lshtm.ac.uk/pmbu/ crf/updated_embl.htm. Brendan Wren's group at the Sanger Institute in collaboration with the Pathogen Sequencing Unit (30/11/2006, revision date)
[138] Hakkinen, M. and Schneitz, C. (1999) Efficacy of a commercial competitive exclusion product against *Campylobacter jejuni*. *Brit. Poult. Sci,* 40, 619-621.
[139] Hald, B., Pedersen, K., Waino, M., Jorgensen, J.C. and Madsen, M. (2004) Longitudinal study of the excretion patterns of thermophilic *Campylobacter* spp. in young pet dogs in Denmark. *J. Clin. Microbiol,* 42, 2003-2012.
[140] Harrington, C.S., Thomson-Carter, F.M. and Carter, P.E. (1997) Evidence of recombination in the flagellin locus of *Campylobacter jejuni*: implications for the flagellin gene typing sheme. *J. Clin. Microbiol,* 35, 2386-2392.
[141] Harris, A.G., Hinds, F.E., Beckhouse, A.G., Kolesnikow, T. and Hazell, S.L. (2002) Resistance to hydrogen peroxide in *Helicobacter pylori*: role of catalase (KatA) and Fur, and functional analysis of a novel gene product designated 'KatA-associated protein', KapA (HP0874). *Microbiology,* 148, 3813-3825.
[142] Harris, A.G. and Hazell, S.L. (2003) Localisation of *Helicobacter pylori* catalase in both the periplasm and cytoplasm, and its dependence on the twin-arginine target protein, KapA, for activity. *FEMS Microbiol. Lett,* 229, 283-289.

[143] Harris, N.V., Weiss, N.S. and Nolan, C.M. (1986) The role of poultry and meats in the etiology of *Campylobacter jejuni/coli* enteritis. *Am. J. Public Health*, 76, 407-411.
[144] Harvey, P. and Leach, S. (1998) Analysis of coccal cell formation by *Campylobacter jejuni* using continuous culture techniques, and the importance of oxidative stress. *J. Appl. Microbiol*, 85, 398-404.
[145] Harvey, R.B., Young, C.R., Anderson, R.C., Droleskey, R.E., Genovese, K.J., Egan, L.F. and Nisbet, D.J. (2000) Diminution of *Campylobacter* colonization in neonatal pigs reared off-sow. *J. Food Prot*, 63, 1430-1432.
[146] Hazel, J.R., Williams, E.E., Livermore, R. and Mozingo, N. (1991) Thermal adaptation in biological membranes: functional significance of changes in phospholipid molecular species composition. *Lipids*, 26, 277-282.
[147] Hazeleger, W.C., Janse, J.D., Koenraad, P.M., Beumer, R.R., Rombouts, F.M. and Abee, T. (1995) Temperature-dependent membrane fatty acid and cell physiology changes in coccoid forms of *Campylobacter jejuni*. *Appl. Environ. Microbiol*, 61, 2713-2719.
[148] Hazeleger, W.C., Wouters, J.A., Rombouts, F.M. and Abee, T. (1998) Physiological Activity of *Campylobacter jejuni* Far below the Minimal Growth Temperature. *Appl. Environ. Microbiol*, 64, 3917-3922.
[149] Hazell, S.L., Evans, D.J., Jr. and Graham, D.Y. (1991) *Helicobacter pylori* catalase. *J. Gen. Microbiol*, 137, 57-61.
[150] Heath, R.J., White, S.W. and Rock, C.O. (2001) Lipid biosynthesis as a target for antibacterial agents. *Progr. Lipid Res*, 40, 467-497.
[151] Heipieper, H.J., Diefenbach, R. and Keweloh, H. (1992) Conversion of cis unsaturated fatty acids to trans, a possible mechanism for the protection of phenol-degrading *Pseudomonas putida* P8 from substrate toxicity. *Appl. Environ. Microbiol*, 58, 1847-1852.
[152] Hendrix, R.W., Smith, M.C., Burns, R.N., Ford, M.E. and Hatfull, G.F. (1999) Evolutionary relationships among diverse bacteriophages and prophages: all the world's a phage. *Proc. Natl. Acad. Sci. USA*, 96, 2192-2197.
[153] Hendrixson, D.R., Akerley, B.J. and DiRita, V.J. (2001) Transposon mutagenesis of *Campylobacter jejuni* identifies a bipartite energy taxis system required for motility. *Mol. Microbiol*, 40, 214-224.

[154] Hendrixson, D.R. and DiRita, V.J. (2003) Transcription of sigma 54-dependent but not sigma 28-dependent flagellar genes in *Campylobacter jejuni* is associated with formation of the flagellar secretory apparatus. *Mol. Microbiol,* 50, 687-702.

[155] Hendrixson, D.R. (2006) A phase-variable mechanism controlling the *Campylobacter jejuni* FlgR response regulator influences commensalism. *Mol. Microbiol,* 61, 1646-1659.

[156] Herren, C.D., Rocha, E.R. and Smith, C.J. (2003) Genetic analysis of an important oxidative stress locus in the anaerobe *Bacteroides fragilis*. *Gene,* 316, 167-175.

[157] Heuer, O.E., Pedersen, K., Andersen, J.S. and Madsen, M. (2001) Prevalence and antimicrobial susceptibility of thermophilic *Campylobacter* in organic and conventional broiler flocks. *Lett. Appl. Microbiol,* 33, 269-274.

[158] Hinton, A., Jr., Cason, J.A., Hume, M.E. and Ingram, K.D. (2004) Use of MIDI-fatty acid methyl ester analysis to monitor the transmission of *Campylobacter* during commercial poultry processing. *J. Food Prot,* 67, 1610-1616.

[159] Hofreuter, D., Tsai, J., Watson, R.O., Novik, V., Altman, B., Benitez, M., Clark, C., Perbost, C., Jarvie, T., Du, L. and Galan, J.E. (2006) Unique features of a highly pathogenic *Campylobacter jejuni* strain. *Infect. Immun,* 74, 4694-4707.

[160] Holler, C., Witthuhn, D. and Janzen-Blunck, B. (1998) Effect of low temperatures on growth, structure, and metabolism of *Campylobacter coli* SP10. *Appl. Environ. Microbiol,* 64, 581- 587.

[161] Hou, Y.M. (1999) Transfer RNAs and pathogenicity islands. *Trends Biomed. Sci,* 24, 295-298.

[162] Hugdhal, M.B., Beery, J.T. and Doyle, M.P. (1988) Chemotactic behavior of *Campylobacter jejuni*. *Infect. Immun,* 56, 1560-1566.

[163] Hutchinson, D.N., Bolton, F.J., Hinchliffe, P.M., Dawkins, H.C., Horsley, S.D., Jessop, E.G., Robertshaw, P.A. and Counter, D.E. (1985) Evidence of udder excretion of *Campylobacter jejuni* as the cause of milk-borne campylobacter outbreak. *J. Hyg.* (Lond.), 94, 205-215.

[164] ICMSF (International commission of Microbiological Specification for Foods). Micro-organisms in food. *Characteristics of microbial pathogens.* (1996) B. Academic, London, United Kingdom, 45-65. Available from:

[165] Ikram, R., Chambers, S., Mitchell, P., Brieseman, M.A. and Ikam, O.H. (1994) A case control study to determine risk factors for campylobacter infection in Christchurch in the summer of 1992-3. *N Z Med. J,* 107, 430-432.
[166] Inglis, G.D., Kalischuk, L.D. and Busz, H.W. (2004) Chronic shedding of *Campylobacter* species in beef cattle. *J. Appl. Microbiol,* 97, 410-420.
[167] Jackowski, S. and Rock, C.O. (1987) Acetoacetyl-acyl carrier protein synthase, a potential regulator of fatty acid biosynthesis in bacteria. *J. Biol. Chem,* 262, 7927-7931.
[168] Jackson, R.J., Elvers, K.T., Lee, L.J., Gidley, M.D., Wainwright, L.M., Lightfoot, J., Park, S.F. and Poole, R.K. (2006) Oxygen reactivity of both respiratory oxidases in *Campylobacter jejuni:* the "cydAB" genes encode a cyanide-resistant, low-affinity oxidase that is not of the cytochrome bd-type. *J. Bacteriol, JB.*00897-06.
[169] Jacob, J., Martin, W. and Holler, C. (1993) Characterization of viable but nonculturable stage of *C. coli,* characterized with respect to electron microscopic findings, whole cell protein and lipooligosaccharide (LOS) patterns. *Zentralbl. Mikrobiol,* 148, 3-10.
[170] Jagannathan, A., Constantinidou, C. and Penn, C.W. (2001) Roles of rpoN, fliA, and flgR in Expression of Flagella in *Campylobacter jejuni. J. Bacteriol,* 183, 2937-2942.
[171] Jagannathan, A. and Penn, C.W. (2005) Motility. In: J.M. Ketley and M.E. Konkel (Eds.). Campylobacter : Molecular and Cellular Biology. Norfolk: *Horizon Bioscience;* 331-347.
[172] Jean, D., Briolat, V. and Reysset, G. (2004) Oxidative stress response in *Clostridium perfringens. Microbiology,* 150, 1649-1659.
[173] Jesse, T.W., Pittenger-Alley, L.G. and Englen, M.D. (2006) Sequence analysis of two cryptic plasmids from an agricultural isolate of *Campylobacter coli. Plasmid,* 55, 64-69.
[174] Jones, D.M., Sutcliffe, E.M. and Curry, A. (1991) Recovery of viable but non-culturable *Campylobacter jejuni. J. Gen. Microbiol,* 137, 2477-2482.
[175] Jones, K. (2001) The *Campylobacter* conundrum. *Trends Microbiol,* 9, 365-366.
[176] Joshua, G.W., Guthrie-Irons, C., Karlyshev, A.V. and Wren, B.W. (2006) Biofilm formation in *Campylobacter jejuni. Microbiology,* 152, 387-396.
[177] Joux, F. and Lebaron, P. (2000) Use of fluorescent probes to assess physiological functions of bacteria at single-cell level. *Microbes Infect,* 2, 1523-1535.

[178] Juven, B.J. and Kanner, J. (1986) Effect of ascorbic, isoascorbic and dehydroascorbic acids on the growth and survival of *Campylobacter jejuni. J. Appl. Bacteriol*, 61, 339-345.

[179] Kalmokoff, M., Lanthier, P., Tremblay, T.L., Foss, M., Lau, P.C., Sanders, G., Austin, J., Kelly, J. and Szymanski, C.M. (2006) Proteomic analysis of *Campylobacter jejuni* 11168 biofilms reveals a role for the motility complex in biofilm formation. *J. Bacteriol*, 188, 4312-4320.

[180] Kanehisa, M. (1997) A database for post-genome analysis. *Trends Genet*, 13, 375-376.

[181] Kapperud, G., Skjerve, E., Bean, N.H., Ostroff, S.M. and Lassen, J. (1992) Risk factors for sporadic *Campylobacter* infections: results of a case-control study in southeastern Norway. *J. Clin. Microbiol*, 30, 3117-3121.

[182] Kapperud, G., Espeland, G., Wahl, E., Walde, A., Herikstad, H., Gustavsen, S., Tveit, I., Natas, O., Bevanger, L. and Digranes, A. (2003) Factors associated with increased and decreased risk of *Campylobacter* infection: a prospective case-control study in Norway. *Am. J. Epidemiol*, 158, 234-242.

[183] Karlyshev, A.V., McCrossan, M.V. and Wren, B.W. (2001) Demonstration of Polysaccharide Capsule in Campylobacter jejuni Using Electron Microscopy. *Infect. Immun*, 69, 5921-5924.

[184] Karlyshev, A.V., Linton, D., Gregson, N.A. and Wren, B.W. (2002) A novel paralogous gene family involved in phase-variable flagella-mediated motility in *Campylobacter jejuni. Microbiology*, 148, 473-480.

[185] Karlyshev, A.V., Ketley, J.M. and Wren, B.W. (2005) The *Campylobacter jejuni* glycome. *FEMS Microbiol. Rev*, 29, 377-390.

[186] KEGG - Fatty acid biosynthesis - *Campylobacter jejuni* NCTC11168 [online]. [Last accessed on 17/01/07]. Available from: http://www.genome.jp/dbget-bin/get_pathway? org_name=cje and mapno=00061. (10/6/05, revision date)

[187] Kelana, L.C. and Griffiths, M.W. (2003) Use of an Autobioluminescent *Campylobacter jejuni* To Monitor Cell Survival as a Function of Temperature, pH, and Sodium Chloride. *J. Food Prot*, 66, 2032-2037.

[188] Kelley, W.L. (2006) Lex marks the spot: the virulent side of SOS and a closer look at the LexA regulon. *Mol. Microbiol*, 62, 1228-1338.

[189] Kelly, A.F., Park, S.F., Bovill, R. and Mackey, B.M. (2001) Survival of *Campylobacter jejuni* during stationary phase: evidence for the absence of a phenotypic stationary-phase response. *Appl. Environ. Microbiol*, 67, 2248-2254.

[190] Kelly, D.J. (2005) Metabolism, electron transport and bioenergetics of *Campylobacter jejuni*: implications for understanding life in the gut and survival in the environment. In: J. Ketley and M.E. Konkel (Eds.). *Campylobacter jejuni*: Molecular and Cellular biology. Norfolk (United Kingdom): *Horizon Bioscience;* 275-292.

[191] Keyer, K., Gort, A.S. and Imlay, J.A. (1995) Superoxide and the production of oxidative DNA damage. *J. Bacteriol*, 177, 6782-6790.

[192] Khakhria, R. and Lior, H. (1992) Extended phage-typing scheme for *Campylobacter jejuni* and *Campylobacter coli*. *Epidemiol. Infect*, 108, 403-414.

[193] Khalil, K., Lindblom, G.B., Mazhar, K., Sjogren, E. and Kaijser, B. (1993) Frequency and enterotoxigenicity of *Campylobacter jejuni* and *C. coli* in domestic animals in Pakistan as compared to Sweden. *J. Trop. Med. Hyg*, 96, 35-40.

[194] Kirov, S.M., Castrisios, M. and Shaw, J.G. (2004) *Aeromonas* flagella (polar and lateral) are enterocyte adhesins that contribute to biofilm formation on surfaces. *Infect. Immun*, 72, 1939-1945.

[195] Kobayashi, N., Nishino, K. and Yamaguchi, A. (2001) Novel macrolide-specific ABC-type efflux transporter in *Escherichia coli*. *J. Bacteriol*, 183, 5639-5644.

[196] Kogure, K., Simidu, U. and Taga, N. (1979) A tentative direct microscopic method for counting living marine bacteria. *Can. J. Microbiol*, 25, 415-420.

[197] Konkel, M.E., Kim, B.J., Klena, J.D., Young, C.R. and Ziprin, R. (1998) Characterization of the thermal stress response of *Campylobacter jejuni*. *Infect. Immun*, 66, 3666-3672.

[198] Krieg, N.R. and Hoffman, P.S. (1986) Microaerophily and oxygen toxicity. *Annu. Rev. Microbiol*, 40, 107-130.

[199] Kumar, A. and Schweizer, H.P. (2005) Bacterial resistance to antibiotics: active efflux and reduced uptake. *Adv. Drug Deliv. Rev*, 57, 1486-1513.

[200] Kuroda, A., Murphy, H., Cashel, M. and Kornberg, A. (1997) Guanosine tetra- and pentaphosphate promote accumulation of inorganic polyphosphate in *Escherichia coli*. *J. Biol. Chem*, 272, 21240-21243.

[201] Kusumaningrum, H.D., van Asselt, E.D., Beumer, R.R. and Zwietering, M.H. (2004) A quantitative analysis of cross-contamination of *Salmonella* and *Campylobacter* spp. via domestic kitchen surfaces. *J. Food Prot*, 67, 1892-1903.
[202] Kuusi, M., Klemets, P., Miettinen, I., Laaksonen, I., Sarkkinen, H., Hanninen, M.L., Rautelin, H., Kela, E. and Nuorti, J.P. (2004) An outbreak of gastroenteritis from a non-chlorinated community water supply. *J. Epidemiol. Commun. Health*, 58, 273-277.
[203] Lambert, J.D. and Macxy, R.B. (1984) Effect of gamma radiation on *Campylobacter jejuni*. *J. Food Sci*, 49, 665-667.
[204] Lambert, M.A., Patton, C.M., Barrett, T.J. and Moss, C.W. (1987) Differentiation of *Campylobacter* and *Campylobacter*-like organisms by cellular fatty acid composition. *J. Clin. Microbiol*, 25, 706-713.
[205] Lazaro, B., Carcamo, J., Audicana, A., Perales, I. and Fernandez-Astroga, A. (1999) Viability and DNA maintenance in nonculturable spiral *Campylobacter jejuni* cells after long-term exposure to low temperatures. *Appl. Environ. Microbiol*, 65, 4677-4681.
[206] Leach, S., Harvey, P. and Wali, R. (1997) Changes with growth rate in the membrane lipid composition of and amino acid utilization by continuous cultures of *Campylobacter jejuni*. *J. Appl. Microbiol*, 82, 631-640.
[207] Lee, A., O'Rourke, J.L., Barrington, P.J. and Trust, T.J. (1986) Mucus colonization as a determinant of pathogenicity in intestinal infection by *Campylobacter jejuni* : a mouse cecal model. *Infect. Immun*, 51, 536-546.
[208] Lee, J.W. and Helmann, J.D. (2006) The PerR transcription factor senses H2O2 by metal-catalysed histidine oxidation. *Nature*, 440, 363-367.
[209] Lee, M.D. and Newell, D.G. (2006) *Campylobacter* in poultry: filling an ecological niche. *Avian Dis*, 50, 1-9.
[210] Lee, M.K., Billington, S.J. and Joens, L.A. (2004) Potential virulence and antimicrobial susceptibility of *Campylobacter jejuni* isolates from food and companion animals. *Foodborne Pathog. Dis*, 1, 223-230.
[211] Lee, Y.-D., Moon, B.-Y., Choi, J.-P., Chang, H.-G., Noh, B.-S. and Park, J.-H. (2005) Isolation, Identification, and Characterization of Aero-Adaptive *Campylobacter jejuni*. *J. Microbiol. Biotechnol*, 15, 992-1000.
[212] Lehtola, M.J., Pitkanen, T., Miebach, L. and Miettinen, I.T. (2006) Survival of *Campylobacter jejuni* in potable water biofilms: a comparative study with different detection methods. *Water Sci. Technol*, 54, 57-61.
[213] Levy, A.J. (1946) A gastro-enteritis outbreak probably due to a bovine strain of *Vibrio*. *Yale J. Biol. Med*, 18, 243-258.

[214] Lewis, S.J., Velasquez, A., Cuppett, S.L. and McKee, S.R. (2002) Effect of electron beam irradiation on poultry meat safety and quality. *Poult. Sci,* 81, 896-903.

[215] Lin, J., Michel, L.O. and Zhang, Q. (2002) CmeABC functions as a multidrug efflux system in *Campylobacter jejuni*. *Antimicrob Agents Chemother,* 46, 2124-2131.

[216] Lin, J., Sahin, O., Michel, L.O. and Zhang, Q. (2003) Critical role of multidrug efflux pump CmeABC in bile resistance and *in vivo* colonization of *Campylobacter jejuni*. *Infect. Immun,* 71, 4250-4259.

[217] Lin, J., Akiba, M. and Zhang, Q. (2005) Multidrug efflux systems in *Campylobacter*. In: J.M. Ketley and M.E. Konkel (Eds.). *Campylobacter*: molecular and cellular biology. Norfolk: *Horizon Bioscience;* 205-218.

[218] Lin, J., Cagliero, C., Guo, B., Barton, Y.W., Maurel, M.C., Payot, S. and Zhang, Q. (2005) Bile salts modulate expression of the CmeABC multidrug efflux pump in *Campylobacter jejuni*. *J. Bacteriol,* 187, 7417-7424.

[219] Lin, J. and Martinez, A. (2006) Effect of efflux pump inhibitors on bile resistance and in vivo colonization of *Campylobacter jejuni*. *J. Antimicrob. Chemother,* 58, 966-972.

[220] Lior, H., Woodward, D.L., Edgar, J.A., Laroche, L.J. and Gill, P. (1982) Serotyping of *Campylobacter jejuni* by slide agglutination based on heat-labile antigenic factors. *J. Clin. Microbiol,* 15, 761-768.

[221] Loc Carrillo, C., Atterbury, R.J., el-Shibiny, A., Connerton, P.L., Dillon, E., Scott, A. and Connerton, I.F. (2005) Bacteriophage therapy to reduce *Campylobacter jejuni* colonization of broiler chickens. *Appl. Environ. Microbiol,* 71, 6554-6563.

[222] Loewen, P.C. and Switala, J. (1987) Multiple catalases in *Bacillus subtilis*. *J. Bacteriol,* 169, 3601-3607.

[223] Loewen, P.C., Carpena, X., Rovira, C., Ivancich, A., Perez-Luque, R., Haas, R., Odenbreit, S., Nicholls, P. and Fita, I. (2004) Structure of *Helicobacter pylori* catalase, with and without formic acid bound, at 1.6 A resolution. *Biochemistry,* 43, 3089-3103.

[224] Luber, P. and Bartelt, E. (2007) Enumeration of *Campylobacter* spp. on the surface and within chicken breast fillets. *J. Appl. Microbiol,* 102, 313-318.

[225] Lumppio, H.L., Shenvi, N.V., Summers, A.O., Voordouw, G. and Kurtz, D.M., Jr. (2001) Rubrerythrin and rubredoxin oxidoreductase in *Desulfovibrio vulgaris*: a novel oxidative stress protection system. *J. Bacteriol*, 183, 101-108.

[226] Luo, N. and Zhang, Q. (2001) Molecular characterization of a cryptic plasmid from *Campylobacter jejuni*. *Plasmid*, 45, 127-133.

[227] Luo, N., Sahin, O., Lin, J., Michel, L.O. and Zhang, Q. (2003) In vivo selection of *Campylobacter* isolates with high levels of fluoroquinolone resistance associated with *gyrA* mutations and the function of the CmeABC efflux pump. *Antimicrob. Agents Chemother*, 47, 390-394.

[228] MacKichan, J.K., Gaynor, E.C., Chang, C., Cawthraw, S., Newell, D.G., Miller, J.F. and Falkow, S. (2004) The *Campylobacter jejuni* dccRS two-component system is required for optimal in vivo colonization but is dispensable for in vitro growth. *Mol. Microbiol*, 54, 1269-1286.

[229] Macnab, R.M. (2003) How bacteria assemble flagella. *Annu. Rev. Microbiol*, 57, 77-100.

[230] Mamelli, L., Amoros, J.P., Pages, J.M. and Bolla, J.M. (2003) A phenylalanine-arginine beta-naphthylamide sensitive multidrug efflux pump involved in intrinsic and acquired resistance of *Campylobacter* to macrolides. *Int. J. Antimicrob. Agents*, 22, 237-241.

[231] Mamelli, L., Prouzet-Mauléon, V., Pages, J.M., Mégraud, F. and Bolla, J.M. (2005) Molecular basis of macrolide resistance in *Campylobacter*: role of efflux pumps and target mutations. *J. Antimicrob. Chemother*, 56, 491-497.

[232] Mamelli, L., Demoulin, E., Prouzet-Mauleon, V., Megraud, F., Pages, J.M. and Bolla, J.M. (2007) Prevalence of efflux activity in low-level macrolide-resistant *Campylobacter* species. *J. Antimicrob. Chemother*, in press.

[233] Manning, G., Dowson, C.G., Bagnall, M.C., Ahmed, I.H., West, M. and Newell, D.G. (2003) Multilocus sequence typing for comparison of veterinary and human isolates of *Campylobacter jejuni*. *Appl. Environ. Microbiol*, 69, 6370-6379.

[234] Marchant, J., Henderson, J., Wren, B.W. and Ketley, J. (1998) Role of the CheY gene in the chemotaxis of *Campylobacter jejuni*. In: A. Lastovica, D. Newell and E. Lastovica (Eds.). *Campylobacter, Helicobacter and Related Organisms*. Cape Town: University of Cape Town; 306-311.

[235] Marchant, J., Wren, B. and Ketley, J. (2002) Exploiting genome sequence: predictions for mechanisms of *Campylobacter* chemotaxis. *Trends Microbiol*, 10, 155-159.

[236] Marrakchi, H., Choi, K.H. and Rock, C.O. (2002) A new mechanism for anaerobic unsaturated fatty acid formation in *Streptococcus pneumoniae*. *J. Biol. Chem*, 277, 44809-44816.

[237] Martinac, B., Adler, J. and Kung, C. (1990) Mechanosensitive ion channels of *E. coli* activated by amphipaths. *Nature*, 348, 261-263.

[238] Martinez, A. and Lin, J. (2006) Effect of an efflux pump inhibitor on the function of the multidrug efflux pump CmeABC and antimicrobial resistance in *Campylobacter*. *Foodborne Pathog. Dis*, 3, 393-402.

[239] Martinez-Rodriguez, A., Kelly, A.F., Park, S.F. and Mackey, B.M. (2004) Emergence of variants with altered survival properties in stationary phase cultures of *Campylobacter jejuni*. *Int. J. Food Microbiol*, 90, 321-329.

[240] Martinez-Rodriguez, A. and Mackey, B.M. (2005) Physiological changes in *Campylobacter jejuni* on entry into stationary phase. *Int. J. Food Microbiol*, 101, 1-8.

[241] Masse, E. and Gottesman, S. (2002) A small RNA regulates the expression of genes involved in iron metabolism in *Escherichia coli*. *Proc. Natl. Acad. Sci. USA*, 99, 4620-4625.

[242] McFadyean, J. and Stockman, S.HMSO (1913) Report of the Departmental Committee appointed by the Board of Agriculture and Fisheries to inquire into epizootic abortion. Part III. Abortion in sheep. London.

[243] McGovern, K.J., Blanchard, T.G., Gutierrez, J.A., Czinn, S.J., Krakowka, S. and Youngman, P. (2001) gamma-Glutamyltransferase is a *Helicobacter pylori* virulence factor but is not essential for colonization. *Infect. Immun*, 69, 4168-4173.

[244] McLaggan, D., Naprstek, J., Buurman, E.T. and Epstein, W. (1994) Interdependence of K+ and glutamate accumulation during osmotic adaptation of *Escherichia coli*. *J. Biol. Chem*, 269, 1911-1917.

[245] McSweegan, E. and Walker, R.I. (1986) Identification and characterization of two *Campylobacter jejuni* adhesins for cellular and mucous substrates. *Infect. Immun*, 53, 141-148.

[246] Medema, G.J., Schets, F.M., van de Giessen, A.W. and Havelaar, A.H. (1992) Lack of colonization of 1 day old chicks by viable, non-culturable *Campylobacter jejuni*. *J. Appl. Bacteriol*, 72, 512-516.

[247] Megli, F.M. and Sabatini, K. (2004) Mitochondrial phospholipid bilayer structure is ruined after liver oxidative injury in vivo. *FEBS Lett,* 573, 68-72.
[248] Meldrum, R.J., Tucker, D. and Edwards, C. (2004) Baseline rates of *Campylobacter* and *Salmonella* in raw chicken in Wales, United Kingdom, in 2002. *J. Food Prot,* 67, 1226-1228.
[249] MIDI, I. (2002) MIS operating manual.Sherlock microbial identification system. 4.5. MIDI, I., Newark.
[250] Miller, W.G. and Mandrell, R.E. (2004) *Campylobacter* in the food and water supply: Prevalence, outbreaks, isolation, and detection. In: J. Ketley and M.E. Konkel (Eds.). *Campylobacter jejuni: New perspectives in molecular and cellular biology.* Norfolk (United Kingdom): Horizon Scientific Press; 109-163.
[251] Mills, S.D., Kuzniar, B., Shames, B., Kurjanczyk, L.A. and Penner, J.L. (1992) Variation of the O antigen of *Campylobacter jejuni* in vivo. *J. Med. Microbiol,* 36, 215-219.
[252] Misra, H.S., Khairnar, N.P., Barik, A., Indira Priyadarsini, K., Mohan, H. and Apte, S.K. (2004) Pyrroloquinoline-quinone: a reactive oxygen species scavenger in bacteria. *FEBS Lett,* 578, 26-30.
[253] MMWR. Morbidity and Mortality Weekly Report. Preliminary FoodNet Data on the Incidence of Infection with Pathogens Transmitted Commonly Through Food --- 10 States, United States, 2005 [online]. [Last accessed on 16/01/07]. Available from: http://www.cdc.gov/mmwr/preview/mmwrhtml/mm5514a2.htm. MMWR Weekly (13/4/2006, revision date) 55 (14), 392-395
[254] Moen, B., Oust, A., Langsrud, O., Dorrell, N., Marsden, G.L., Hinds, J., Kohler, A., Wren, B.W. and Rudi, K. (2005) Explorative multifactor approach for investigating global survival mechanisms of *Campylobacter jejuni* under environmental conditions. *Appl. Environ. Microbiol,* 71, 2086-2094.
[255] Mohammed, K.A., Miles, R.J. and Halablab, M.A. (2004) The pattern and kinetics of substrate metabolism of *Campylobacter jejuni* and *Campylobacter coli. Lett. Appl. Microbiol,* 39, 261-266.
[256] Mohan, S., Kelly, T.M., Eveland, S.S., Raetz, C.R. and Anderson, M.S. (1994) An *Escherichia coli* gene (FabZ) encoding (3R)-hydroxymyristoyl acyl carrier protein dehydrase. Relation to fabA and suppression of mutations in lipid A biosynthesis. *J. Biol. Chem,* 269, 32896-32903.

[257] Moran, A.P. and Upton, M.E. (1987) Effect of medium supplements, illumination and superoxide dismutase on the production of coccoid forms of *Campylobacter jejuni* ATCC 29428. *J. Appl. Bacteriol,* 62, 43-51.

[258] Moran, A.P. and Penner, J.L. (1999) Serotyping of *Campylobacter jejuni* based on heat-stable antigens: relevance, molecular basis and implications in pathogenesis. *J. Appl. Microbiol,* 86, 361-377.

[259] Moran, A.P., Penner, J.L. and Aspinall, G.O. (2000) *Campylobacter* lipolysaccharides. In: I. Nachamkin and M.J. Blaser (Eds.). *Campylobacter.* Washington, D.C.: ASM Press; 241-257.

[260] Morgan, G.J., Hatfull, G.F., Casjens, S. and Hendrix, R.W. (2002) Bacteriophage Mu genome sequence: analysis and comparison with Mu-like prophages in *Haemophilus, Neisseria* and *Deinococcus. J. Mol. Biol,* 317, 337-359.

[261] Moss, C.W., Kai, A., Lambert, M.A. and Patton, C. (1984) Isoprenoid quinone content and cellular fatty acid composition of *Campylobacter* species. *J. Clin. Microbiol,* 19, 772-776.

[262] Mouery, K., Rader, B.A., Gaynor, E.C. and Guillemin, K. (2006) The stringent response is required for *Helicobacter pylori* survival of stationary phase, exposure to acid, and aerobic shock. *J. Bacteriol,* 188, 5494-5500.

[263] Murphy, C., Carroll, C. and Jordan, K.N. (2003) Induction of an adaptive tolerance response in the foodborne pathogen, *Campylobacter jejuni. FEMS Microbiol. Lett,* 223, 89-93.

[264] Murphy, C., Carroll, C. and Jordan, K.N. (2003) Identification of a novel stress resistance mechanism in *Campylobacter jejuni. J. Appl. Microbiol,* 95, 704-708.

[265] Murphy, C., Carroll, C. and Jordan, K.N. (2006) Environmental survival mechanisms of the foodborne pathogen *Campylobacter jejuni. J. Appl. Microbiol,* 100, 623-632.

[266] Murphy, P., Dowds, B.C., McConnell, D.J. and Devine, K.M. (1987) Oxidative stress and growth temperature in *Bacillus subtilis. J. Bacteriol,* 169, 5766-5770.

[267] Naess, V. and Hofstad, T. (1984) Chemical composition and biological activity of lipopolysaccharides prepared from type strains of *Campylobacter jejuni* and *Campolybacter coli. Acta Pathol. Microbiol. Immunol. Scand.* [B], 92, 217-222.

[268] Narberhaus, F. (1999) Negative regulation of bacterial heat shock genes. *Mol. Microbiol,* 31, 1-8.

[269] Neimann, J., Engberg, J., Molbak, K. and Wegener, H.C. (2003) A case-control study of risk factors for sporadic campylobacter infections in Denmark. *Epidemiol. Infect,* 130, 353-366.
[270] Newell, D.G., McBride, H. and Pearson, A.D. (1984) The identification of outer membrane proteins and flagella of *Campylobacter jejuni. J. Gen. Microbiol,* 130, 1201-1208.
[271] Newell, D.G. and Davison, H. (2003) *Campylobacter* control and prevention. In: M.E. Torrence and R.E. Isaacson (Eds.). *Microbial Food Safety in Animal Agriculture. Current Topics.* Ames, USA: Iowa State Press; 211-220.
[272] Newell, D.G. and Fearnley, C. (2003) Sources of *Campylobacter* colonization in broiler chickens. *Appl. Environ. Microbiol,* 69, 4343-4351.
[273] Nguyen, H.T.T., Corry, J.E.L. and Miles, C.A. (2006) Heat Resistance and Mechanism of Heat Inactivation in Thermophilic Campylobacters. *Appl. Environ. Microbiol,* 72, 908-913.
[274] Nichols, D.S., Nichols, P.D. and McMeekin, T.A. (1993) Polyunsaturated fatty acids in Antarctic bacteria. *Antarct. Sci,* 5, 144-160.
[275] Nichols, G.L. (2005) Fly transmission of *Campylobacter. Emerg. Infect. Dis,* 11, 361-364.
[276] Nielsen, E.M. (2002) Occurrence and strain diversity of thermophilic campylobacters in cattle of different age groups in dairy herds. *Lett. Appl. Microbiol,* 35, 85-89.
[277] Nikaido, H. (2003) Molecular basis of bacterial outer membrane permeability revisited. *Microbiol. Mol. Biol. Rev,* 67, 593-656.
[278] Nilsson, H.O., Blom, J., Abu-Al-Soud, W., Ljungh, A.A., Andersen, L.P. and Wadstrom, T. (2002) Effect of cold starvation, acid stress, and nutrients on metabolic activity of *Helicobacter pylori. Appl. Environ. Microbiol,* 68, 11-19.
[279] Nirdnoy, W., Mason, C.J. and Guerry, P. (2005) Mosaic structure of a multiple-drug-resistant, conjugative plasmid from *Campylobacter jejuni. Antimicrob. Agents Chemother,* 49, 2454-2459.
[280] Nishino, K., Latifi, T. and Groisman, E.A. (2006) Virulence and drug resistance roles of multidrug efflux systems of *Salmonella enterica* serovar Typhimurium. *Mol. Microbiol,* 59, 126-141.

[281] Obiri-Danso, K., Paul, N. and Jones, K. (2001) The effects of UVB and temperature on the survival of natural populations and pure cultures of *Campylobacter jejuni*, Camp. coli, Camp. lari and urease-positive thermophilic campylobacters (UPTC) in surface waters. *J. Appl. Microbiol,* 90, 256-267.

[282] O'Brien, D.K. and Melville, S.B. (2000) The anaerobic pathogen *Clostridium perfringens* can escape the phagosome of macrophages under aerobic conditions. *Cell Microbiol,* 2, 505-519.

[283] Omidbakhsh, N. (2006) A new peroxide-based flexible endoscope-compatible high-level disinfectant. *Am. J. Infect. Control,* 34, 571-577.

[284] O'Toole, G.A. and Kolter, R. (1998) Initiation of biofilm formation in *Pseudomonas fluorescens* WCS365 proceeds via multiple, convergent signalling pathways: a genetic analysis. *Mol. Microbiol,* 28, 449-461.

[285] Oust, A., Moen, B., Martens, H., Rudi, K., Naes, T., Kirschner, C. and Kohler, A. (2006) Analysis of covariance patterns in gene expression data and FT-IR spectra. *J. Microbiol. Meth,* 65, 573-584.

[286] Pages, J.M. (2004) Bacterial porin and antibiotic susceptibility. *Médecine - Sciences.* (Paris), 20, 346-351.

[287] Palyada, K., Threadgill, D. and Stintzi, A. (2004) Iron acquisition and regulation in *Campylobacter jejuni*. *J. Bacteriol,* 186, 4714-4729.

[288] Park, A.M., Li, Q., Nagata, K., Tamura, T., Shimono, K., Sato, E.F. and Inoue, M. (2004) Oxygen tension regulates reactive oxygen generation and mutation of *Helicobacter pylori*. *Free Radic. Biol. Med,* 36, 1126-1133.

[289] Park, S., You, X. and Imlay, J.A. (2005) Substantial DNA damage from submicromolar intracellular hydrogen peroxide detected in Hpx- mutants of *Escherichia coli*. *Proc. Natl. Acad. Sci. USA,* 102, 9317-9322.

[290] Park, S.F. (2000) Environmental regulatory genes. In: I. Nachamkin and M.J. Blaser (Eds.). *Campylobacter*, 2nd edition. Washington DC: ASM press; 423-440.

[291] Park, S.F. (2002) The physiology of *Campylobacter* species and its relevance to their role as foodborne pathogens. *Int. J. Food Microbiol,* 74, 177-188.

[292] Park, S.F. (2005) *Campylobacter jejuni* stress responses during survival in the food chain and colonisation. In: J. Ketley and M.E. Konkel (Eds.). *Campylobacter jejuni*: Molecular and Cellular biology. Norfolk (United Kingdom): *Horizon Bioscience;* 275-292.

[293] Parker, C.T., Quinones, B., Miller, W.G., Horn, S.T. and Mandrell, R.E. (2006) Comparative genomic analysis of *Campylobacter jejuni* strains reveals diversity due to genomic elements similar to those present in *C. jejuni* strain RM1221. *J. Clin. Microbiol,* 44, 4125-4135.

[294] Parkhill, J., Wren, B.W., Mungall, K., Ketley, J.M., Churcher, C., Basham, D., Chillingworth, T., Davies, R.M., Feltwell, T., Holroyd, S., Jagels, K., Karlyshev, A.V., Moule, S., Pallen, M.J., Penn, C.W., Quail, M.A., Rajandream, M.A., Rutherford, K.M., van Vliet, A.H., Whitehead, S. and Barrell, B.G. (2000) The genome sequence of the food-borne pathogen *Campylobacter jejuni* reveals hypervariable sequences. *Nature,* 403, 665-668.

[295] Payot, S., Cloeckaert, A. and Chaslus-Dancla, E. (2002) Selection and characterization of fluoroquinolone-resistant mutants of *Campylobacter jejuni* using enrofloxacin. *Microb. Drug Resist,* 8, 335-343.

[296] Payot, S., Avrain, L., Magras, C., Praud, K., Cloeckaert, A. and Chaslus-Dancla, E. (2004) Relative contribution of target gene mutation and efflux to fluoroquinolone and erythromycin resistance, in French poultry and pig isolates of *Campylobacter coli*. *Int. J. Antimicrob. Agents,* 23, 468-472.

[297] Payot, S., Bolla, J.M., Corcoran, D., Fanning, S., Megraud, F. and Zhang, Q. (2006) Mechanisms of fluoroquinolone and macrolide resistance in *Campylobacter* spp. *Microbes Infect,* 8, 1967-1971.

[298] Pearson, A.D., Greenwood, M., Healing, D., Rollins, D., Shahamat, M., Donaldson, J. and Colwell, R.R. (1993) Colonization of broiler chickens by waterbone *Campylobacter jejuni*. *Appl. Environ. Microbiol,* 59, 987-996.

[299] Pearson, B.M., Pin, C., Wright, J., I'Anson, K., Humphrey, T. and Wells, J.M. (2003) Comparative genome analysis of *Campylobacter jejuni* using whole genome DNA microarrays. *FEBS Lett,* 554, 224-230.

[300] Penner, J.L., Pearson, A.D. and Hennessy, J.N. (1983) Investigation of a waterborne outbreak of *Campylobacter jejuni* enteritis with a serotyping scheme based on thermostable antigens. *J. Clin. Microbiol.* .18, 1362-1365.

[301] Pesci, E.C., Cottle, D.L. and Pickett, C.L. (1994) Genetic, enzymatic, and pathogenic studies of the iron superoxide dismutase of *Campylobacter jejuni*. *Infect. Immun,* 62, 2687-2694.

[302] Pesci, E.C. and Pickett, C.L. (1994) Genetic organization and enzymatic activity of a superoxide dismutase from the microaerophilic human pathogen, *Helicobacter pylori*. *Gene,* 143, 111-116.

[303] Poly, F., Threadgill, D. and Stintzi, A. (2004) Identification of *Campylobacter jejuni* ATCC 43431-specific genes by whole microbial genome comparisons. *J. Bacteriol,* 186, 4781-4795.

[304] Poole, K. (2005) Efflux-mediated antimicrobial resistance. *J. Antimicrob. Chemother,* 56, 20-51.

[305] Primm, T.P., Andersen, S.J., Mizrahi, V., Avarbock, D., Rubin, H. and Barry, C.E., 3rd. (2000) The stringent response of *Mycobacterium tuberculosis* is required for long-term survival. *J. Bacteriol,* 182, 4889-4898.

[306] Prouty, M.G., Correa, N.E. and Klose, K.E. (2001) The novel sigma54- and sigma28-dependent flagellar gene transcription hierarchy of *Vibrio cholerae. Mol. Microbiol,* 39, 1595-1609.

[307] Pumbwe, L. and Piddock, L.J. (2002) Identification and molecular characterisation of CmeB, a *Campylobacter jejuni* multidrug efflux pump. *FEMS Microbiol. Lett,* 206, 185-189.

[308] Pumbwe, L., Randall, L.P., Woodward, M.J. and Piddock, L.J. (2004) Expression of the efflux pump genes *cmeB, cmeF* and the porin gene *porA* in multiple-antibiotic-resistant *Campylobacter jejuni. J. Antimicrob. Chemother,* 54, 341-347.

[309] Pumbwe, L., Randall, L.P., Woodward, M.J. and Piddock, L.J. (2005) Evidence for multiple-antibiotic resistance in *Campylobacter jejuni* not mediated by CmeB or CmeF. *Antimicrob. Agents Chemother,* 49, 1289-1293.

[310] Quinn, T., Bolla, J.M., Pages, J.M. and Fanning, S. (2007) Antibiotic-resistant *Campylobacter*: could efflux pump inhibitors control infection? *J. Antimicrob. Chemother, in press.*

[311] Ramarao, N., Gray-Owen, S.D. and Meyer, T.F. (2000) *Helicobacter pylori* induces but survives the extracellular release of oxygen radicals from professional phagocytes using its catalase activity. *Mol. Microbiol,* 38, 103-113.

[312] Raphael, B.H., Pereira, S., Flom, G.A., Zhang, Q., Ketley, J.M. and Konkel, M.E. (2005) The *Campylobacter jejuni* Response Regulator, CbrR, Modulates Sodium Deoxycholate Resistance and Chicken Colonization. *J. Bacteriol,* 187, 3662-3670.

[313] Ratledge, C. and Wilkinson, S.G. (1988) Fatty acids, related and derived lipids. In: C. Ratledge and S.G. Wilkinson (Eds.). *Microbial lipids.* London, United Kingdom: Academic Press; 23-52.

[314] Reischl, S., Wiegert, T. and Schumann, W. (2002) Isolation and Analysis of Mutant Alleles of the *Bacillus subtilis* HrcA Repressor with Reduced Dependency on GroE Function. *J. Biol. Chem*, 277, 32659-32667.

[315] Rocha, E.R., Selby, T., Coleman, J.P. and Smith, C.J. (1996) Oxidative stress response in an anaerobe, *Bacteroides fragilis*: a role for catalase in protection against hydrogen peroxide. *J. Bacteriol*, 178, 6895-6903.

[316] Rocha, E.R., Herren, C.D., Smalley, D.J. and Smith, C.J. (2003) The complex oxidative stress response of *Bacteroides fragilis*: the role of OxyR in control of gene expression. *Anaerobe*, 9, 165-173.

[317] Rock, C.O. and Jackowski, S. (2002) Forty years of bacterial fatty acid synthesis. *Biochem. Biophys. Res. Comm*, 292, 1155-66.

[318] Rodriguez, G.G., Phipps, D., Ishiguro, K. and Ridgway, H.F. (1992) Use of a fluorescent redox probe for direct visualization of actively respiring bacteria. *Appl. Environ. Microbiol*, 58, 1801-1808.

[319] Rollins, D.M. and Colwell, R.R. (1986) Viable but nonculturable stage of *Campylobacter jejuni* and its role in survival in the natural aquatic environment. *Appl. Environ. Microbiol*, 52, 531-538.

[320] Romeo, T. (1998) Global regulation by the small RNA-binding protein CsrA and the non-coding RNA molecule CsrB. *Mol. Microbiol*, 29, 1321-1330.

[321] Rosario, M.M., Fredrick, K.L., Ordal, G.W. and Helmann, J.D. (1994) Chemotaxis in *Bacillus subtilis* requires either of two functionally redundant CheW homologs. *J. Bacteriol*, 176, 2736-2739.

[322] Rosenquist, H., Nielsen, N.L., Sommer, H.M., Norrung, B. and Christensen, B.B. (2003) Quantitative risk assessment of human campylobacteriosis associated with thermophilic *Campylobacter* species in chickens. *Int. J. Food Microbiol*, 83, 87-103.

[323] Roszak, D.B. and Colwell, R.R. (1987) Metabolic activity of bacterial cells enumerated by direct viable count. *Appl. Environ. Microbiol*, 53, 2889-2893.

[324] Russell, N.J. (1984) Mechanisms of thermal adaptation in bacteria : blueprints for survival. *Trends Biomed. Sci*, 9, 108-112.

[325] Russell, N.J. (1989) Functions of lipids: structural roles in membrane functions. In: C. Ratledge and S.G. Wilkinson (Eds.). *Microbial lipids*. Toronto, Canada: Academic Press; 279-365.

[326] Russell, N.J. and Fukunaga, N. (1990) A comparison of thermal adaptation of membrane lipids in psychrophilic and thermophilic bacteria. *FEMS Microbiol. Rev*, 75, 171-182.

[327] Russell, N.J., (1995). Psychrotrophy and adaptation to low temperatures: microbial membrane lipids. Proceedings of the 19th International congress on Refrigeration. Workshop Refrigeration and Microbiology: Health, Food, Drinks and Flowers, pp. 359-365.

[328] Russell, N.J., Evans, R.I., ter Steeg, P.F., Hellemons, J., Verheul, A. and Abee, T. (1995) Membranes as a target for stress adaptation. *Int. J. Food Microbiol,* 28, 255-261.

[329] Saha, S.K., Saha, S. and Sanyal, S.C. (1991) Recovery of injured *Campylobacter jejuni* cells after animal passage. *Appl. Environ. Microbiol,* 57, 3388-3389.

[330] Sahin, O., Luo, N., Huang, S. and Zhang, Q. (2003) Effect of *Campylobacter*-specific maternal antibodies on *Campylobacter jejuni* colonization in young chickens. *Appl. Environ. Microbiol,* 69, 5372-5379.

[331] Sails, A.D., Swaminathan, B. and Fields, P.I. (2003) Utility of multilocus sequence typing as an epidemiological tool for investigation of outbreaks of gastroenteritis caused by *Campylobacter jejuni. J. Clin. Microbiol,* 41, 4733-9.

[332] Sajbidor, J. (1997) Effect of some environmental factors on the content and composition of microbial membrane lipids. *Crit. Rev. Biotechnol,* 17, 87-103.

[333] Salama, S.M., Bolton, F.J. and Hutchinson, D.N. (1990) Application of a new phagetyping scheme to campylobacters isolated during outbreaks. *Epidemiol. Infect,* 104, 405-11.

[334] Salloway, S., Mermel, L.A., Seamans, M., Aspinall, G.O., Nam Shin, J.E., Kurjanczyk, L.A. and Penner, J.L. (1996) Miller-Fisher syndrome associated with *Campylobacter jejuni* bearing lipopolysaccharide molecules that mimic human ganglioside GD3. *Infect. Immun,* 64, 2945-2949.

[335] Sampathkumar, B., Napper, S., Carillo, C., Willson, P., Taboada, E., Nash, J.H.E., Potter, A.A., Babiuk, L.A. and Allan, B.J. (2006) Transcriptional and translational expression patterns associated with immobilized growth of *Campylobacter jejuni. Microbiology,* 152, 567-577.

[336] The Sanger Centre - *Campylobacter jejuni* [online]. [Last accessed on 18/01/2007]. Available from: http://www.sanger.ac.uk/Projects/C_jejuni. (15/01/2007, revision date)

[337] Schoeni, J.L. and Doyle, M.P. (1992) Reduction of *Campylobacter jejuni* colonization of chicks by cecum-colonizing bacteria producing anti-*C. jejuni* metabolites. *Appl. Environ. Microbiol,* 58, 664-70.
[338] Schorr, D., Schmid, H., Rieder, H.L., Baumgartner, A., Vorkauf, H. and Burnens, A. (1994) Risk factors for *Campylobacter* enteritis in Switzerland. *Zentralbl. Hyg.Umweltmed.,* 196, 327-37.
[339] Schwerer, B., Neisser, A.R., Polt, J., Bernheimer, H. and Moran, A.P. (1995) Antibody cross-reactivities between gangliosides and lipopolysaccharides of *Campylobacter jejuni* serotypes associated with Guillain-Barre´ syndrome. *J. Endotoxin. Res,* 2, 395-403.
[340] Scott, M.D., Meshnick, S.R. and Eaton, J.W. (1987) Superoxide dismutase-rich bacteria. Paradoxical increase in oxidant toxicity. *J. Biol. Chem,* 262, 3640-3645.
[341] Sebald, M. and Veron, M. (1963) Base DNA Content and Classification of Vibrios. *Ann. Inst. Pasteur.* (Paris), 105, 897-910.
[342] Seltmann, G. and Holst, O. (2002) The bacterial cell wall. Berlin, Heidelberg, Germany: Springer.
[343] Sinensky, M. (1974) Homeoviscous adaptation--a homeostatic process that regulates the viscosity of membrane lipids in *Escherichia coli. Proc. Natl. Acad. Sci. USA,* 71, 522-525.
[344] Skelly, C. and Weinstein, P. (2003) Pathogen survival trajectories: an eco-environmental approach to the modeling of human campylobacteriosis ecology. *Environ. Health Persp,* 111, 19-28.
[345] Skorko-Glonek, J., Zurawa, D., Kuczwara, E., Wozniak, M., Wypych, Z. and Lipinska, B. (1999) The *Escherichia coli* heat shock protease HtrA participates in defense against oxidative stress. *Mol. Gen. Genet,* 262, 342-350.
[346] Slavik, F.M., Kim, J.W., Pharr, M.D., Raben, D.P., Tsai, S. and Lobs, C.M. (1994) Effect of trisodium phosphate on *Campylobacter* attached to post-chill chicken carcasses. *J. Food Prot,* 57, 324-326.
[347] Sleator, R.D. and Hill, C. (2002) Bacterial osmoadaptation: the role of osmolytes in bacterial stress and virulence. *FEMS Microbiol. Rev,* 26, 49-71.
[348] Snelling, W.J., McKenna, J.P., Lecky, D.M. and Dooley, J.S. (2005) Survival of *Campylobacter jejuni* in waterborne protozoa. *Appl. Environ. Microbiol,* 71, 5560-5571.
[349] Solomon, E.B. and Hoover, D.G. (2004) Inactivation of *Campylobacter jejuni* by high hydrostatic pressure. *Lett. Appl. Microbiol,* 38, 505-9.

[350] Somers, E.B., Schoeni, J.L. and Wong, A.C.L. (1994) Effect of trisodium phosphate on biofilm and planktonic cells of *Campylobacter jejuni*, *Escherichia coli* O157:H7, *Listeria monocytogenes* and *Salmonella typhimurium*. *Int. J. Food Microbiol*, 22, 269-276.

[351] Sommerlad, S.M. and Hendrixson, D.R. (2007) Analysis of the roles of FlgP and FlgQ in flagellar motility of *Campylobacter jejuni*. *J. Bacteriol*, 189, 179-186.

[352] Sorqvist, S. (2003) Heat resistance in liquids of Enterococcus spp., Listeria spp., Escherichia coli, Yersinia enterocolitica, Salmonella spp. and Campylobacter spp. Acta Vet. Scand, 44, 1-19.

[353] Spohn, G. and Scarlato, V. (1999) Motility of *Helicobacter pylori* is coordinately regulated by the transcriptional activator FlgR, an NtrC homolog. *J. Bacteriol*, 181, 593-599.

[354] Spohn, G., Danielli, A., Roncarati, D., Delany, I., Rappuoli, R. and Scarlato, V. (2004) Dual Control of *Helicobacter pylori* Heat Shock Gene Transcription by HspR and HrcA. *J. Bacteriol*, 186, 2956-2965.

[355] Stanley, K.N., Wallace, J.S., Currie, J.E., Diggle, P.J. and Jones, K. (1998) The seasonal variation of thermophilic campylobacters in beef cattle, dairy cattle and calves. *J. Appl. Microbiol*, 85, 472-480.

[356] Stead, D. and Park, S.F. (2000) Roles of Fe superoxide dismutase and catalase in resistance of *Campylobacter coli* to freeze-thaw stress. *Appl. Environ. Microbiol*, 66, 3110-3112.

[357] Steele, M., McNab, B., Fruhner, L., DeGrandis, S., Woodward, D. and Odumeru, J.A. (1998) Epidemiological Typing of *Campylobacter* Isolates from Meat Processing Plants by Pulsed-Field Gel Electrophoresis, Fatty Acid Profile Typing, Serotyping, and Biotyping. *Appl. Environ. Microbiol*, 64, 2346-2349.

[358] Stern, N.J., Clavero, M.R., Bailey, J.S., Cox, N.A. and Robach, M.C. (1995) *Campylobacter* spp. in broilers on the farm and after transport. *Poult. Sci*, 74, 937-941.

[359] Stern, N.J., Svetoch, E.A., Eruslanov, B.V., Kovalev, Y.N., Volodina, L.I., Perelygin, V.V., Mitsevich, E.V., Mitsevich, I.P. and Levchuk, V.P. (2005) *Paenibacillus polymyxa* purified bacteriocin to control *Campylobacter jejuni* in chickens. *J. Food Prot*, 68, 1450-1453.

[360] Stern, N.J., Svetoch, E.A., Eruslanov, B.V., Perelygin, V.V., Mitsevich, E.V., Mitsevich, I.P., Pokhilenko, V.D., Levchuk, V.P., Svetoch, O.E. and Seal, B.S. (2006) Isolation of a *Lactobacillus salivarius* strain and purification of its bacteriocin, which is inhibitory to *Campylobacter jejuni* in the chicken gastrointestinal system. *Antimicrob. Agents Chemother,* 50, 3111-6.

[361] Stintzi, A. (2003) Gene Expression Profile of *Campylobacter jejuni* in Response to Growth Temperature Variation. *J. Bacteriol,* 185, 2009-2016.

[362] Stock, A.M., Robinson, V.L. and Goudreau, P.N. (2000) Two-Component Signal Transduction. *Annu. Rev. Biochem,* 69, 183-215.

[363] Storz, G. and Imlay, J.A. (1999) Oxidative stress. *Curr. Opin. Microbiol,* 2, 188-194.

[364] Studahl, A. and Andersson, Y. (2000) Risk factors for indigenous campylobacter infection: a Swedish case-control study. *Epidemiol. Infect,* 125, 269-275.

[365] Suerbaum, S., Josenhans, C., Sterzenbach, T., Drescher, B., Brandt, P., Bell, M., Droge, M., Fartmann, B., Fischer, H.P., Ge, Z., Horster, A., Holland, R., Klein, K., Konig, J., Macko, L., Mendz, G.L., Nyakatura, G., Schauer, D.B., Shen, Z., Weber, J., Frosch, M. and Fox, J.G. (2003) The complete genome sequence of the carcinogenic bacterium *Helicobacter hepaticus*. *Proc. Natl. Acad. Sci. USA,* 100, 7901-7906.

[366] Sung, K., Hiett, K.L. and Stern, N.J. (2005) Heat-treated *Campylobacter* spp. and mRNA stability as determined by reverse transcriptase-polymerase chain reaction. *Foodborne Pathog. Dis,* 2, 130-137.

[367] Suutari, M. and Laakso, S. (1992) Temperature adaptation in *Lactobacillus fermentum*: interconversions of oleic, vaccenic and dihydrosterulic acids. *J. Gen. Microbiol,* 138, 445-450.

[368] Szurmant, H. and Ordal, G.W. (2004) Diversity in Chemotaxis Mechanisms among the Bacteria and Archaea. *Microbiol. Mol. Biol. Rev,* 68, 301-319.

[369] Szymanski, C.M., Michael, F.S., Jarrell, H.C., Li, J., Gilbert, M., Larocque, S., Vinogradov, E. and Brisson, J.R. (2003) Detection of conserved N-linked glycans and phase-variable lipooligosaccharides and capsules from *Campylobacter* cells by mass spectrometry and high resolution magic angle spinning NMR spectroscopy. *J. Biol. Chem,* 278, 24509-24520.

[370] Taboada, E.N., Acedillo, R.R., Carrillo, C.D., Findlay, W.A., Medeiros, D.T., Mykytczuk, O.L., Roberts, M.J., Valencia, C.A., Farber, J.M. and Nash, J.H. (2004) Large-scale comparative genomics meta-analysis of *Campylobacter jejuni* isolates reveals low level of genome plasticity. *J. Clin. Microbiol,* 42, 4566-4576.

[371] Talibart, R., Denis, M., Castillo, A., Cappelier, J.M. and Ermel, G. (2000) Survival and recovery of viable but noncultivable forms of *Campylobacter* in aqueous microcosm. *Int. J. Food Microbiol,* 55, 263-267.

[372] Tam le, T., Antelmann, H., Eymann, C., Albrecht, D., Bernhardt, J. and Hecker, M. (2006) Proteome signatures for stress and starvation in *Bacillus subtilis* as revealed by a 2-D gel image color coding approach. *Proteomics,* 6, 4565-4585.

[373] Tatchou-Nyamsi-Konig, J.-A., Moreau, A., Federighi, M. and Block, J.-C. (OnlineEarly Articles) Behaviour of *Campylobacter jejuni* in experimentally contaminated bottled natural mineral water. *J. Appl. Microbiol.*

[374] Taylor, D.E., Garner, R.S. and Allan, B.J. (1983) Characterization of tetracycline resistance plasmids from *Campylobacter jejuni* and *Campylobacter coli*. *Antimicrob. Agents Chemother,* 24, 930-935.

[375] Taylor, D.E. and Tracz, D.M. (2005) Mechanisms of antimicrobial resistance in *Campylobacter*. In: J.M. Ketley and M.E. Konkel (Eds.). *Campylobacter*: molecular and cellular biology. Norfolk: Horizon Bioscience; 193-204.

[376] Tenover, F.C., Williams, S., Gordon, K.P., Nolan, C. and Plorde, J.J. (1985) Survey of plasmids and resistance factors in *Campylobacter jejuni* and *Campylobacter coli*. *Antimicrob. Agents Chemother,* 27, 37-41.

[377] Thackray, P.D. and Moir, A. (2003) SigM, an extracytoplasmic function sigma factor of *Bacillus subtilis*, is activated in response to cell wall antibiotics, ethanol, heat, acid, and superoxide stress. *J. Bacteriol,* 185, 3491-3498.

[378] Tholozan, J.L., Cappelier, J.M., Tissier, J.P., Delattre, G. and Federighi, M. (1999) Physiological characterization of viable-but-nonculturable *Campylobacter jejuni* cells. *Appl. Environ. Microbiol,* 65, 1110-1116.

[379] Thomas, C., Hill, D.J. and Mabey, M. (1999) Morphological changes of synchronized *Campylobacter jejuni* populations during growth in single phase liquid culture. *Lett. Appl. Microbiol,* 28, 194-198.

[380] Thomas, C., Hill, D. and Mabey, M. (2002) Culturability, injury and morphological dynamics of thermophilic *Campylobacter* spp. within a laboratory-based aquatic model system. *J. Appl. Microbiol,* 92, 433-442.

[381] Tomb, J.-F., White, O., Kerlavage, A.R., Clayton, R.A., Sutton, G.G., Fleischmann, R.D., Ketchum, K.A., Klenk, H.P., Gill, S., Dougherty, B.A., Nelson, K., Quackenbush, J., Zhou, L., Kirkness, E.F., Peterson, S., Loftus, B., Richardson, D., Dodson, R., Khalak, H.G., Glodek, A., McKenney, K., Fitzegerald, L.M., Lee, N., Adams, M.D., Hickey, E.K., Berg, D.E., Gocayne, J.D., Utterback, T.R., Peterson, J.D., Kelley, J.M., Cotton, M.D., Weidman, J.M., Fujii, C., Bowman, C., Watthey, L., Wallin, E., Hayes, W.S., Borodovsky, M., Karp, P.D., Smith, H.O., Fraser, C.M. and Venter, J.C. (1997) The complete genome sequence of the gastric pathogen *Helicobacter pylori*. *Nature,* 388, 539-547.

[382] Trachoo, N. and Franck, J.F. (2002) Effectiveness of chemical sanitizers against *Campylobacter jejuni*-contaning biofilms. *J. Food Prot,* 65, 1117-1121.

[383] Trachoo, N., Franck, J.F. and Stern, N.J. (2002) Survival of *Campylobacter jejuni* in biofilms isolated from chicken houses. *J. Food Prot,* 65, 1110-1116.

[384] Unden, G. (1999) Aerobic respiration and regulation of aerobic/anaerobic metabolism. In: J.W. Lengeler, G. Drews and H.G. Schlegel (Eds.). *Biology of the prokaryotes.* New-York, Thieme, Stuttgart: Blackwell Science.

[385] Urban, C.F., Lourido, S. and Zychlinsky, A. (2006) How do microbes evade neutrophil killing? *Cell Microbiol,* 8, 1687-1696.

[386] Vaara, M. (1992) Agents that increase the permeability of the outer membrane. *Microbiol. Rev,* 56, 395-411.

[387] van Vliet, A.H., Wooldridge, K.G. and Ketley, J.M. (1998) Iron-responsive gene regulation in a *Campylobacter jejuni* fur mutant. *J. Bacteriol,* 180, 5291-5298.

[388] van Vliet, A.H.M., Baillon, M.-L.A., Penn, C.W. and Ketley, J.M. (2001) The iron-induced ferredoxin FdxA of *Campylobacter jejuni* is involved in aerotolerance. *FEMS Microbiol. Lett,* 196, 189-193.

[389] Van Vliet, A.H.M., Ketley, J.M., Park, S.F. and Penn, C.W. (2002) The role of iron in *Campylobacter* gene regulation, metabolism and oxidative stress defense. *FEMS Microbiol. Rev,* 26, 173-186.

[390] Vatanyoopaisarn, S., Nazli, A., Dodd, E., Rees, C.E. and Waites, W.M. (2002) Effect of flagella on initial attachment of *Listeria monocytogenes* to stainless steel. *Appl. Environ. Microbiol,* 66, 860-863.

[391] Vellinga, A. and Van Loock, F. (2002) The dioxin crisis as experiment to determine poultry-related campylobacter enteritis. *Emerg. Infect. Dis,* 8, 19-22.

[392] Wagenaar, J.A., Mevius, D.J. and Havelaar, A.H. (2006) *Campylobacter* in primary animal production and control strategies to reduce the burden of human campylobacteriosis. *Rev. Sci. Technol,* 25, 581-594.

[393] Wagner, D., Maser, J., Lai, B., Cai, Z., Barry, C.E., 3rd, Honer Zu Bentrup, K., Russell, D.G. and Bermudez, L.E. (2005) Elemental analysis of *Mycobacterium avium-, Mycobacterium tuberculosis-,* and *Mycobacterium smegmatis-*containing phagosomes indicates pathogen-induced microenvironments within the host cell's endosomal system. *J. Immunol,* 174, 1491-1500.

[394] Wai, S.N., Nakayama, K., Umene, K., Moriya, T. and Amako, K. (1996) Construction of a ferritin-deficient mutant of *Campylobacter jejuni*: contribution of ferritin to iron storage and protection against oxidative stress. *Mol. Microbiol,* 20, 1127-1134.

[395] Wait, R. and Hudson, M.J. (1985) The use of picolinyl esters for the characterization of microbial lipids: application to the unsaturated and cyclopropane fatty acids of *Campylobacter* species. *Lett. Appl. Microbiol,* 1, 95-99.

[396] Wang, A.Y. and Cronan, J.E., Jr. (1994) The growth phase-dependent synthesis of cyclopropane fatty acids in *Escherichia coli* is the result of an RpoS(KatF)-dependent promoter plus enzyme instability. *Mol. Microbiol,* 11, 1009-1017.

[397] Wang, G., Alamuri, P. and Maier, R.J. (2006) The diverse antioxidant systems of *Helicobacter pylori. Mol. Microbiol,* 61, 847-860.

[398] Wang, H. and Cronan, J.E. (2004) Functional replacement of the FabA and FabB proteins of *Escherichia coli* fatty acid synthesis by Enterococcus faecalis FabZ and FabF homologues. *J. Biol. Chem,* 279, 34489-34495.

[399] Wareing, D.R., Bolton, F.J., Fox, A.J., Wright, P.A. and Greenway, D.L. (2002) Phenotypic diversity of *Campylobacter* isolates from sporadic cases of human enteritis in the UK. *J. Appl. Microbiol,* 92, 502-509.

[400] Wassenaar, T.M., van der Zeijst, B.A., Ayling, R. and Newell, D.G. (1993) Colonization of chicks by motility mutants of *Campylobacter jejuni* demonstrates the importance of flagellin A expression. *J. Gen. Microbiol*, 139 Pt 6, 1171-1175.

[401] Wassenaar, T.M. and Newell, D.G. (2000) Genotyping of *Campylobacter* spp. *Appl. Environ. Microbiol*, 66, 1-9.

[402] Waterman, S.R., Hackett, J. and Manning, P.A. (1993) Characterization of the replication region of the small cryptic plasmid of *Campylobacter hyointestinalis*. *Gene*, 125, 11-17.

[403] Waterman, S.R. and Small, P.L. (1998) Acid-sensitive enteric pathogens are protected from killing under extremely acidic conditions of pH 2.5 when they are inoculated onto certain solid food sources. *Appl. Environ. Microbiol*, 64, 3882-3886.

[404] Williams, G.M. and Jeffrey, A.M. (2000) Oxidative DNA damage: endogenous and chemically induced. *Regular Toxicol. Pharmacol*, 32, 283-292.

[405] Wolfe, A.J., Chang, D.E., Walker, J.D., Seitz-Partridge, J.E., Vidaurri, M.D., Lange, C.F., Prüss, B.M., Henk, M.C., Larkin, J.C. and Conway, T. (2003) Evidence that acetyl phosphate functions as a global signal during biofilm development. *Mol. Microbiol*, 48, 977-988.

[406] Wosten, M.M., Parker, C.T., van Mourik, A., Guilhabert, M.R., van Dijk, L. and van Putten, J.P. (2006) The *Campylobacter jejuni* PhosS/PhosR operon represents a non-classical phosphate-sensitive two-component system. *Mol. Microbiol*, 62, 278-291.

[407] Wosten, M.M.S.M., Wagenaar, J.A. and van Putten, J.P.M. (2004) The FlgS/FlgR Two-component Signal Transduction System Regulates the fla Regulon in *Campylobacter jejuni*. *J. Biol. Chem*, 279, 16214-16222.

[408] Wu, Y.L., Lee, L.H., Rollins, D.M. and Ching, W.M. (1994) Heat shock and alkaline pH-induced proteins of *Campylobacter jejuni* : Characterization and immunological properties. *Infect. Immun*, 62, 4256-4260.

[409] Yamanaka, K., Fang, L. and Inouye, M. (1998) The CspA family in *Escherichia coli*: multiple gene duplication for stress adaptation. *Mol. Microbiol*, 27, 247-255.

[410] Yamasaki, M., Igimi, S., Katayama, Y., Yamamoto, S. and Amano, F. (2004) Identification of an oxidative stress-sensitive protein from *Campylobacter jejuni*, homologous to rubredoxin oxidoreductase/rubrerythrin. *FEMS Microbiol. Lett*, 235, 57-63.

[411] Yan, M., Sahin, O., Lin, J. and Zhang, Q. (2006) Role of the CmeABC efflux pump in the emergence of fluoroquinolone-resistant *Campylobacter* under selection pressure. *J. Antimicrob. Chemother,* 58, 1154-1159.

[412] Yao, R., Burr, D.H. and Guerry, P. (1997) CheY-mediated modulation of *Campylobacter jejuni* virulence. *Mol. Microbiol,* 23, 1021-1031.

[413] Zambrano, M.M., Siegele, D.A., Almiron, M., Tormo, A. and Kolter, R. (1993) Microbial competition: *Escherichia coli* mutants that take over stationary phase cultures. *Science,* 259, 1757-1760.

[414] Zhang, W., Brooun, A., McCandless, J., Banda, P. and Alam, M. (1996) Signal transduction in the Archaeon *Halobacterium salinarium* is processed through three subfamilies of 13 soluble and membrane-bound transducer proteins. *Proc. Natl. Acad. Sci. USA,* 93, 4649-4654.

[415] Zhao, T. and Doyle, M.P. (2006) Reduction of *Campylobacter jejuni* on chicken wings by chemical treatments. *J. Food Prot,* 69, 762-767.

[416] Zheng, M., Wang, X., Templeton, L.J., Smulski, D.R., LaRossa, R.A. and Storz, G. (2001) DNA microarray-mediated transcriptional profiling of the *Escherichia coli* response to hydrogen peroxide. *J. Bacteriol,* 183, 4562-4570.

[417] Zinser, E.R. and Kolter, R. (2000) Prolonged stationary-phase incubation selects for lrp mutations in *Escherichia coli* K-12. *J. Bacteriol,* 182, 4361-4365.

[418] Zoonoses Report - United Kingdom 2004 [online] Department for Environment, Food and Rural Affairs (2005) London, United Kingdom, Available from: http://www.defra.gov.uk/animalh/diseases/zoonoses/zoonoses_reports/zoonoses 2004.pdf.

Index

A

abdominal, 1
abortion, 3, 17, 117
acceptor (s), 33, 44, 49
access, 87
acetate, 7
acid, 14, 25, 29, 42, 43, 44, 47, 48, 56, 57, 58, 65, 68, 69, 70, 71, 72, 73, 74, 75, 77, 79, 89, 96, 101, 102, 108, 109, 110, 111, 112, 114, 115, 117, 119, 120, 124, 129, 131
acidic, 65, 132
acquired immunity, 19
actinomycetes, 64
activation, 59, 64, 82, 84
activators, 80
active site, 47, 87, 106
acute, 1
Adams, 130
adaptation, 42, 45, 58, 62, 67, 73, 74, 85, 87, 94, 106, 109, 117, 124, 125, 126, 128, 132
adenosine, 99
adhesion, 96
adult (s), 21, 25
aerobe, 49, 56
aerobic, 44, 46, 50, 52, 58, 60, 61, 93, 119, 121, 130

agar, 51, 90
age, 18, 20, 21, 41, 97, 120
agent (s), 22, 46, 51, 52, 53, 101, 109
agglutination, 115
aggregates, 89
aging, 98
agricultural, 36, 111
aid, 8
air, 12, 39, 46, 47, 50
alcohol (s), 56, 68
aldehydes, 48, 49
alkaline, 132
allele (s), 9, 36
alpha, 63
alternative, 35, 44, 45, 53, 64, 84, 94
ambient air, 46, 50
amines, 47
amino, 29, 44, 47, 57, 65, 81, 87, 96, 114
amino acid (s), 44, 47, 65, 81, 96, 114
aminoglycosides, 77
ammonia, 89
amphoteric, 79
anaerobe (s), 46, 49, 50, 60, 110, 124
anaerobic, 32, 44, 46, 51, 52, 61, 117, 121, 130
animal health, 3
animal models, 32, 83

animals, 5, 10, 17, 18, 19, 20, 21, 22, 23, 39, 61, 102, 113, 114
anion (s), 46, 47, 48, 51, 52, 53
Antarctic, 120
antibacterial agents, 109
antibiotic (s), vii, 10, 44, 46, 58, 68, 77, 78, 79, 80, 81, 82, 93, 104, 113, 121, 123, 129
antibody, 88, 100
antigen, 7, 69, 72, 77, 78, 118
antigenicity, 30
antimicrobial, 25, 81, 82, 95, 110, 114, 117, 123, 129
antioxidant (s), 32, 107, 131
application, 9, 16, 21, 40, 131
aquaporin, 42
aquatic, 100, 124, 130
archaea, 86, 128
arginine, 47, 108, 116
arrest, 63
arthritis, 1
artificial, 14
ascorbic, 14, 112
assessment, 124
assignment, 34
assimilation, 44
asymptomatic, 17, 19
atmosphere, 5, 15, 50, 89
ATP, 61, 63, 68, 76, 79, 91
ATP-binding cassette (ABC), 55, 76, 79, 81, 91, 113
ATPase, 33
attachment, 87, 90, 131
attacks, vii, 53
attribution, 23
atypical, 75, 79
Australia, 97
autoimmune disease (s), 72
availability, 21, 27, 40, 52, 65
avoidance, 11

B

B. subtilis, 30, 50, 51, 53, 54, 55, 56, 57, 58, 59, 60, 63, 64, 82, 85, 86, 87, 93
Bacillus subtilis, 49, 56, 71, 80, 98, 100, 101, 105, 106, 115, 119, 124, 129
bacteria, vii, 3, 9, 11, 12, 14, 15, 16, 22, 36, 40, 42, 43, 44, 45, 46, 50, 51, 52, 53, 57, 58, 59, 62, 63, 64, 65, 67, 68, 69, 71, 72, 73, 75, 76, 77, 78, 79, 80, 82, 83, 86, 88, 100, 104, 107, 108, 111, 113, 116, 118, 120, 124, 126
bacterial, 11, 12, 21, 22, 23, 24, 29, 40, 41, 44, 45, 53, 64, 68, 69, 71, 72, 80, 87, 89, 93, 103, 104, 107, 108, 119, 120, 124, 126
bacterial cells, 71, 124
bacterial strains, 12
bacteriocin, 15, 127, 128
bacteriophage (s), 8, 21, 31, 34, 107, 109
bacteriostatic, 14
bacterium, vii, 1, 5, 39, 41, 43, 44, 45, 49, 51, 62, 69, 78, 82, 83, 87, 93, 128
barrier (s), 20, 65, 67, 79, 82
base pair, 29
beef, 24, 104, 111, 127
behavior, 110
Belgium, 9
beta, 63, 69, 77, 78, 108, 116
bias, 29
bile, 80, 83, 115
binding, 33, 35, 36, 54, 57, 58, 59, 64, 69, 76, 79, 80, 91, 100, 105, 124
biochemical, 6, 7
bioenergetics, 113
biofilm formation, 22, 87, 89, 90, 94, 112, 113, 121
biofilms, 87, 88, 89, 90, 100, 101, 102, 112, 114, 130
biogenesis, 32, 83
biological, 30, 34, 35, 91, 98, 109, 119
biological activity, 119
biological responses, 91

Index

biology, 37, 113, 115, 118, 121, 129
biomolecules, 44, 47
biosecurity, 19, 20
biosynthesis, 29, 32, 33, 34, 44, 68, 69, 70, 71, 78, 102, 109, 111, 112, 118
biosynthetic pathways, 75
birds, 17, 19, 21, 22, 24, 39, 91
birth, 18, 19
blood, 3, 5
bonds, 69
bovine, 114
branching, 73
breakdown, 49
breast, 50, 115
breeding, 11
broilers, 95, 127
buffer, 13
by-products, 49

C

caecum, 20
campylobacter, 18, 19, 20, 22, 23, 24, 95, 110, 111, 120, 128, 131
campylobacter enteritis, 131
Campylobacter jejuni, vii, 1, 3, 4, 5, 6, 11, 13, 16, 21, 27, 29, 30, 35, 39, 40, 41, 42, 45, 49, 50, 61, 65, 71, 73, 79, 80, 81, 86, 95, 96, 97, 98, 99, 100, 101, 102, 103, 104, 105, 106, 107, 108, 109, 110, 111, 112, 113, 114, 115, 116, 117, 118, 119, 120, 121, 122, 123, 124, 125, 126, 127, 128, 129, 130, 131, 132, 133
Campylobacter jejuni infection, 98, 106
Canada, 18, 124
capacity, 22, 25, 35, 61, 62, 83
Cape Town, 116
capsular biosynthesis (CAP), 33
capsule, 7, 31, 34, 62, 89
carbohydrates, 43, 62
carbon, 44, 45, 47, 48, 49, 50, 52, 58, 104
carbon dioxide, 44, 49, 50, 104

carbon-centered radicals, 47
carboxyl, 68, 69
carcinogenesis, 49
carcinogenic, 128
carotenoids, 68
carrier, 69, 70, 108, 111, 118
catabolic, 44
catalase, 6, 52, 54, 56, 57, 58, 60, 61, 62, 98, 101, 103, 108, 109, 115, 123, 124, 127
catalytic, 47, 56
cation (s), 49, 77, 79, 105
cats, 21, 95, 98, 103
cattle, 17, 18, 19, 24, 95, 97, 98, 111, 120, 127
cecum, 15, 126
cell, 1, 5, 14, 34, 36, 42, 43, 45, 46, 49, 51, 56, 58, 59, 60, 62, 63, 67, 68, 73, 76, 77, 81, 87, 89, 90, 95, 109, 111, 126, 129, 131
cell death, 63
cell membranes, 46
certainty, 33
changing environment, 45, 69
channels, 42, 88, 117
chaperones, 61, 63
charcoal, 5
chemical (s), 11, 51, 72, 77, 103, 130, 133
chemoattractants, 86
chemoreceptors, 107
chemotaxis, 34, 83, 85, 86, 90, 116, 117
chicken (s), 9, 10, 12, 15, 16, 19, 20, 21, 24, 45, 50, 63, 80, 83, 88, 98, 99, 101, 103, 104, 105, 115, 118, 120, 122, 124, 125, 126, 127, 128, 130, 133
chicks, 20, 117, 126, 132
children, 3
chloride, 6, 16, 40, 112
chlorination, 24
chlorine, 14, 89
chromosome, 29, 30, 31, 32, 35, 64, 86
ciprofloxacin, 79, 80, 81, 107
cis, 69, 70, 71, 73, 108, 109
classes, 79
classical, 40, 132

Index

classification, 4
classified, 30, 34, 49, 50
cleaning, 14, 20
cleavage, 48
clinical, 37
clones, 104
cloning, 100
clusters, 29, 30, 32, 48, 49
CO_2, 5, 6, 15, 32, 47, 50
codes, 29, 53, 58
coding, 9, 29, 35, 36, 37, 56, 58, 59, 60, 81, 124, 129
codon (s), 35, 36, 80
collaboration, 108
colonisation, 17, 18, 19, 20, 45, 93, 99, 121
colonization, 11, 20, 32, 80, 83, 85, 99, 102, 109, 114, 115, 116, 117, 120, 125, 126
commensalism, 110
commensals, 21
commercial, 24, 72, 108, 110
communication, 24
community, 114
competition, 133
complement, 84
complications, 1
components, 7, 32, 44, 45, 62, 68, 80, 82, 84, 105
composition (s), 41, 43, 58, 67, 71, 72, 73, 74, 75, 76, 78, 102, 109, 114, 119, 125
compounds, 5, 42, 44, 48, 76
computer, 72
concentration, 33, 51, 57, 71, 73, 74, 79
condensation, 41, 70
conditioning, 15, 46
congress, 125
consensus, 35
conservation, 15
construction, 96
consumption, 16, 24, 61, 65
contaminants, 16
contamination, 1, 9, 11, 12, 14, 16, 24, 88, 97, 114
continuing, 61

control, 9, 10, 11, 14, 20, 24, 86, 95, 104, 106, 107, 111, 112, 120, 123, 124, 127, 128, 131
controlled, 45, 59, 78, 80
convex, 6
Copenhagen, 96
correlation, 7, 73, 79, 80, 82
coupling, 82
coverage, 31
cows, 18
CRP, 44
crystalline, 73
C-terminal, 58, 86
cultural, 22
culture, 5, 6, 18, 51, 52, 73, 89, 109, 129
cyanide, 111
cyanobacteria, 69
cycles, 70
cyclopropane Fatty Acids (CFA), 71, 74
cysteine, 43, 47
cytochrome, 32, 33, 44, 59, 60, 111
cytoplasm, 7, 56, 67, 77, 108
cytoplasmic membrane, 36, 67, 76, 77, 82, 103
cytosol, 44, 48
cytosolic, 49

D

dairy, 18, 95, 107, 120, 127
danger, 17
database, 9, 27, 112
death, 22, 63
defense, 126, 130
deficiency, 45
definition, 87
degenerate, 5
degradation, 44, 57
degree, 72
dehydrate, 48
dehydration, 62
dehydrogenases, 44

delivery, 37
denaturation, 63
Denmark, 10, 18, 96, 108, 120
density, 35
dependant, 18, 19, 24, 56
deprivation, 22, 58, 108
derivatives, 96
desiccation, 12
destruction, 14
detection, 40, 100, 101, 114, 118
detergents, 68, 80
detoxification, 46, 49, 50, 53, 59
detoxifying, 5, 58
developing countries, vii, 1
DGGE, 84
diagnostic, 5, 6
diarrhea, 1, 3
diarrhoea, 21
dienes, 47
diffusion, 16, 42, 51, 78, 79
digestive tract, 40, 61
dioxin, 9, 131
discrimination, 8, 9
discriminatory, 23
diseases, 72
Disinfectant, 97
disinfection, 20
distribution, 12
diversity, 31, 32, 41, 86, 95, 104, 120, 122, 131
division, 5, 40, 71, 76, 79
DNA, 8, 23, 29, 30, 31, 32, 33, 34, 35, 36, 40, 47, 49, 53, 54, 57, 58, 62, 63, 64, 84, 97, 113, 114, 121, 122, 126, 132, 133
DNA damage, 47, 53, 57, 58, 113, 121, 132
DNA repair, 30
dogs, 21, 95, 108
donors, 44
double bonds, 69
drinking, 12, 20, 88
drug resistance, 77, 120
drugs, 77, 78, 82
duplication, 132

duration, 14
dyes, 80

E

E. coli, 13, 15, 16, 30, 41, 42, 43, 44, 47, 48, 50, 52, 53, 54, 55, 56, 57, 58, 59, 60, 63, 64, 65, 70, 71, 74, 75, 78, 79, 80, 81, 82, 83, 85, 86, 87, 93, 117
eating, 103
ecological, 19, 22, 114
ecology, 22, 126
ecosystem, 106
efficacy, 11, 15, 82
efflux transporter, 113
elderly, 25
electron, 33, 40, 44, 49, 51, 68, 105, 111, 113, 115
electron beam, 115
electron microscopy, 105
electrophoresis, 23
elongation, 40, 41, 70, 73
emergence, 80, 100, 133
emerging issues, 96
encoding, 30, 32, 33, 36, 41, 57, 59, 62, 63, 78, 81, 82, 84, 90, 118
endogenous, 132
endoscope, 121
endotoxins, 69
energy, 44, 45, 61, 63, 67, 86, 90, 109
England, 88
enteric, 22, 83, 107, 132
enteritis, vii, 1, 10, 22, 23, 93, 102, 103, 109, 114, 122, 126, 131
envelope, 34, 36, 63, 68
environment, 1, 17, 18, 19, 21, 22, 23, 39, 40, 43, 61, 67, 69, 75, 82, 85, 86, 88, 91, 94, 105, 113, 124
environmental, vii, 1, 19, 21, 22, 23, 45, 58, 64, 67, 72, 82, 85, 88, 91, 93, 99, 103, 118, 125, 126
environmental change, 2

environmental conditions, 1, 67, 82, 85, 88, 118
environmental factors, 72, 125
environmental stimuli, 45
environmental threats, 91
enzymatic, 40, 44, 122
enzyme (s), 5, 9, 15, 32, 33, 44, 47, 48, 51, 52, 53, 70, 71, 74, 90, 131
epidemic, 3, 9
epidemiological, 7, 8, 17, 20, 22, 23, 24, 125
epidemiology, 8, 19, 20, 106
epithelial cell (s), 32, 53, 56, 99
equilibrium, 79
equipment, 11, 44
erosion, 88
Escherichia coli, 34, 62, 74, 78, 96, 99, 100, 101, 102, 103, 105, 106, 107, 108, 113, 117, 118, 121, 126, 127, 131, 132, 133
essential oils, 105
ester, 68, 72, 108, 110
esterase, 85
esters, 131
ethanol, 75, 129
ethanolamine, 68
etiology, 109
eukaryotic, 68
Europe, 11
European, 19
evidence, 18, 19, 22, 29, 40, 42, 82, 113
evolution, 9
evolutionary, 24
excitation, 85, 86
exclusion, 21, 108
excretion, 108, 110
exogenous, 56
exotic, 22
exponential, 43, 52, 63, 75
exporter, 79
exposure, 21, 24, 40, 51, 53, 58, 62, 63, 65, 75, 114, 119
external environment, 67
extracellular, 29, 43, 88, 89, 123
extrusion, 76, 79

F

faecal, 18, 19, 22, 24, 85
family, 4, 12, 42, 44, 61, 69, 76, 79, 80, 86, 112, 132
farm (s), 20, 21, 23, 61, 88, 95, 96, 127
farmers, 9, 20
farmland, 106
fatty acid (s), 43, 48, 49, 58, 65, 68, 69, 70, 71, 72, 73, 74, 75, 77, 99, 101, 102, 107, 108, 109, 110, 111, 114, 117, 119, 120, 124, 131
fecal, 3, 20
feces, 3, 10, 32
feedback, 64, 87
feeding, 98
ferritin, 57, 90, 131
fetus, 3, 4, 8, 17, 27, 28, 71, 98, 102
fiber, 89
filament, 83, 90
films, 12
filtration, 97
fish, 10
fitness, 43
flagellum, 5, 7, 83
flexibility, 44, 67
floating, 89
fluid, 67
fluoroquinolones, 25, 77, 78, 80
folding, 63
food, vii, 1, 3, 5, 9, 11, 12, 14, 15, 16, 24, 25, 45, 46, 61, 62, 65, 96, 104, 105, 110, 114, 118, 121, 122, 132
food industry, 11, 16, 46
food poisoning, 1, 3, 16
food products, 15, 16
food safety, 46
foodstuffs, 5, 11, 16
Ford, 109
fowl, 19, 24
Fox, 104, 106, 128, 131
fragility, 18

fragmentation, 47
France, 16
freezing, 12, 62, 75
FT-IR, 121
fumarate, 44
functional analysis, 108
Fur, 45, 54, 55, 58, 59, 60, 100, 108
fusion, 79, 87, 91

G

gamma radiation, 114
gangliosides, 72, 126
gas, 41, 88, 89, 90, 99, 106
gastric, 65, 97, 102, 130
gastric mucosa, 102
gastroenteritis, 3, 39, 114, 125
gastrointestinal, 11, 128
geese, 19
gel, 16, 23, 129
gene (s), 9, 23, 29, 30, 31, 32, 33, 34, 35, 36, 37, 41, 42, 43, 45, 52, 53, 54, 55, 56, 57, 58, 59, 60, 61, 62, 63, 64, 71, 74, 78, 80, 81, 83, 84, 86, 89, 90, 93, 96, 98, 99, 101, 103, 106, 108, 110, 111, 112, 116, 117, 118, 119, 121, 122, 123, 124, 130, 132
gene expression, 61, 63, 64, 84, 96, 121, 124
gene transfer, 34
generation, 61, 85, 121
generators, 51
genetic (s), 9, 21, 22, 23, 41, 57, 81, 104, 121
genetic diversity, 104
genetic information, 57
genetic instability, 23
genome, vii, 1, 9, 21, 23, 27, 28, 29, 30, 31, 33, 34, 36, 37, 42, 44, 53, 56, 61, 62, 63, 64, 74, 76, 80, 81, 83, 86, 87, 93, 94, 104, 106, 108, 112, 117, 119, 122, 123, 128, 129, 130
genome sequences, 1, 21, 53, 93
genome sequencing, 28, 61

genomic (s), 16, 23, 27, 30, 31, 32, 33, 93, 122, 129
genomic regions, 33
Germany, 3, 126
glass, 89
gluconeogenesis, 44
glucose, 43
glutamate, 41, 117
glutamine, 43, 47, 56, 105, 106
glutathione, 32
glycans, 128
glycerol, 33, 68
glycine, 42
glycoconjugates, 72
glycogen, 44
glycolipids, 69
glycolysis, 44
glycoproteins, 52
glycosylation, 32, 57, 89
gracilis, 4
Gram-negative, 5, 15, 39, 62, 64, 68, 69, 71, 72, 75, 76, 78, 79, 104
Gram-positive, 15, 69, 79
granules, 44
grapes, 10
grass, 18
Great Britain, 18
green fluorescent protein, 103
GroEL, 63, 64, 90
grouping, 29
groups, 34, 49, 71, 73, 77, 120
growth, 5, 6, 22, 32, 33, 43, 44, 45, 49, 50, 51, 58, 61, 62, 63, 65, 67, 69, 71, 73, 74, 75, 78, 83, 88, 89, 90, 91, 99, 102, 104, 105, 110, 112, 114, 116, 119, 125, 129, 131
growth rate, 43, 51, 74, 75, 114
growth temperature, 62, 63, 73, 119
guanine, 49
Guillain-Barre syndrome, 1, 72
gut, 17, 18, 19, 45, 113

H

H. pylori, 29, 30, 32, 35, 36, 44, 45, 50, 51, 52, 53, 56, 57, 58, 59, 60, 61, 82, 87, 93
habituation, 99
haemoglobin, 105
handling, 20, 24
Hawaii, 10
head, 68, 73
health, 1, 17, 19, 22, 24, 25, 93, 94
heat, 43, 57, 58, 62, 63, 64, 75, 90, 99, 101, 115, 119, 126, 129
heat shock protein, 63, 64, 90
heating, 13, 14
Helicobacter pylori, vii, 42, 49, 64, 84, 95, 97, 98, 100, 102, 108, 109, 115, 117, 119, 120, 121, 122, 123, 127, 130, 131
helix, 5, 58
heme, 33, 56
heterogeneity, 95
heterogeneous, 4
high pressure, 58
high resolution, 128
high temperature, 1, 12, 40, 74, 78
high-level, 121
histidine, 47, 59, 82, 114
Holland, 128
homeostasis, 58, 59, 67
homolog, 34, 80, 81, 127
homology, 36
homopolymers, 96
horizontal gene transfer, 34
host, 1, 17, 21, 22, 24, 34, 46, 51, 57, 60, 85, 131
hostile environment, 39, 45
household, 9
HSP, 63
human (s), vii, 1, 8, 11, 16, 17, 18, 19, 20, 22, 23, 24, 25, 37, 39, 61, 65, 93, 97, 98, 99, 104, 116, 122, 124, 125, 126, 131
hybrid, 83, 86
hydro, 42, 69, 76, 77, 79
hydrogen peroxide, 43, 46, 51, 52, 53, 56, 58, 59, 60, 101, 108, 121, 124, 133
hydrolysis, 7
hydroperoxides, 56
hydrophilic, 42, 69, 76, 77, 79
hydrophobic, 69, 77, 78, 79
hydrophobicity, 78, 104
hydrostatic pressure, 75, 126
hydroxyl, 46, 47, 48, 49
hygiene, 5, 12, 16
hypothesis, 25, 79

I

ice, 62
identification, 5, 8, 9, 34, 40, 71, 72, 100, 103, 118, 120
identity, 80, 81
Illinois, 3
illumination, 119
immune system, vii
immunity, 20
immunocompromised, 25
immunoglobulin, 69
immunological, 132
in vitro, 16, 25, 41, 59, 80, 83, 85, 100, 105, 116
in vivo, 41, 63, 74, 85, 115, 116, 118
inactivation, 13, 77, 81
inactive, 43
incidence, 11
incubation, 73, 89, 133
indication, 53
indigenous, 95, 128
induction, 34, 63, 65, 91
industrialized countries, 3, 11
industry, 11, 16, 46
ineffectiveness, 23
inert, 89, 91
infants, 107

infection (s), 1, 8, 9, 10, 12, 13, 17, 18, 19, 20, 21, 22, 23, 24, 29, 32, 34, 95, 98, 101, 106, 107, 111, 112, 114, 120, 123, 128
infectious disease, 3
infertility, 17
inhibition, 16
inhibitor (s), 40, 43, 81, 115, 117, 123
inhibitory, 15, 128
initiation, 35, 37
injury (ies), 62, 118, 130
inoculation, 88
inorganic, 44, 113
inositol, 68
insects, 21
insertion, 31, 32
instability, 23, 131
integrases, 34
integration, 34
integrity, 40, 58, 69
interaction (s), 83, 86, 95, 99, 107
interdisciplinary, 101
interface, 2, 89
Internet, 9
interpretation, 22, 75
intervention, 20, 25
intervention strategies, 21
intestinal tract, 2, 17, 39, 80, 85, 91, 93
intestine, 20, 32, 83
intrinsic, 80, 116
ion channels, 117
ionizing radiation, 13
ions, 47, 53, 67, 72
IR spectra, 121
Ireland, 95
iron, 7, 46, 48, 49, 51, 53, 57, 58, 59, 90, 97, 100, 117, 122, 130, 131
irradiation, 13, 115
island, 30, 34
isolation, 3, 22, 118
isomerization, 70
isozyme, 53

J

January, 27, 28
Jordan, 95, 119

K

K^+, 41, 117
K-12, 133
killing, 130, 132
kinase, 82, 84, 85, 86, 87
kinetics, 63, 101, 118
King, 100

L

lactams, 77, 78
Lactobacillus, 15, 128
lactoperoxidase, 15, 98
lamellar, 67
lead, 15, 25, 27, 48, 51, 52
ligands, 86
limitation (s), 45, 63
linkage, 47
lipid (s), 41, 47, 48, 49, 52, 67, 68, 69, 72, 73, 74, 77, 104, 108, 109, 114, 118, 123, 124, 125, 126, 131
lipid peroxidation, 47, 48
lipophilic, 68
lipopolysaccharide (LPS) (s), 7, 8, 68, 69, 72, 76, 77, 78, 79, 82, 96, 97, 106, 119, 125, 126
liquid interfaces, 90
liquid phase, 88
liquids, 127
Listeria monocytogenes, 105, 127, 131
literature, 72
liver, 17, 34, 118
livestock, 11, 16, 17, 18, 20, 22, 24, 104
locus, 33, 34, 85, 108, 110
London, 99, 110, 117, 123, 133
long distance, 46

long period, 17, 46
long-term, 41, 98, 114, 123
low temperatures, 73, 93, 110, 114, 125
low-level, 78, 80, 116
lysine, 47
lysis, 8, 42

M

machines, 11
macromolecules, 63
macrophage (s), 46, 56, 98, 121
maintenance, 11, 41, 68, 90, 114
malondialdehyde, 48
management, 20, 21
manganese, 53, 55
manganese superoxide dismutase, 53
marine mammals, 21
market, 9
mass spectrometry, 128
mastitis, 18, 24
maternal, 20, 125
matrix, 12, 87, 89
maturation, 88
measures, 1, 11, 16, 20, 94
meat, 9, 10, 12, 13, 14, 24, 102, 115
media, 13, 14, 40, 42, 50, 62, 85
medicine, 46
membrane permeability, 79, 120
membranes, 2, 40, 43, 46, 48, 49, 67, 68, 69, 94, 103, 109
menadione, 51
meta-analysis, 129
metabolic, 33, 40, 43, 45, 49, 77, 88, 93, 120
metabolism, 9, 34, 43, 45, 62, 63, 110, 117, 118, 130
metabolites, 2, 15, 126
metal ions, 47
metals, 46
methionine, 47, 57, 95
methyl viologen, 51
methylation, 87
methylene, 71
methyl-accepting chemotaxis proteins (MCP), 86, 87
mice, 32, 83, 102
microaerophilic, vii, 1, 3, 4, 5, 44, 46, 49, 93, 97, 122
microarray, 33, 62, 104, 133
microbes, 3, 111, 122, 130
microbial, 33, 72, 73, 87, 102, 110, 118, 120, 123, 124, 125, 131, 133
microcosm (s), 97, 105, 129
microenvironments, 131
microorganism (s), 1, 3, 4, 5, 11, 12, 16, 46, 49, 50, 51, 52, 53
microscope, 5
microscopy, 89, 105
microwave, 14, 102
milk, 3, 9, 10, 12, 14, 15, 18, 24, 98, 102, 110
mimicry, 72
mineral water, 129
misfolded, 64
mitochondrial membrane, 49
mixing, 11
MnSOD, 53
mobility, 5
model system, 130
modeling, 126
models, 21, 24, 32, 41, 45, 83
modulation, 87, 133
moieties, 49
molecular changes, 41
molecular mimicry, 72
molecular weight, 50, 78
molecules, 16, 42, 63, 68, 72, 77, 78, 79, 88, 125
molybdenum, 33
monomeric, 79
Moon, 114
morphological, 41, 130
mosaic, 6
motion, 87
mouse, 97, 114
movement, 18, 20, 86

mRNA, 61, 63, 128
mucin, 86, 96
mucosa, 102
mucus, 20
multidrug resistance, 76, 79
multiplication, 40
mutagenesis, 81, 109
mutant (s), 21, 32, 43, 51, 56, 57, 58, 63, 64, 80, 81, 83, 84, 96, 90, 100, 105, 107, 121, 122, 130, 131, 132, 133
mutation (s), 23, 43, 77, 80, 81, 89, 90, 100, 105, 107, 116, 118, 121, 122, 133
Mycobacterium, 123, 131

N

N-acety, 72
NaCl (sodium chloride), 5, 6, 16, 42, 83
NAD, 70
NADH, 70
Nash, 101, 125, 129
national, 18, 19, 95
natural, 1, 22, 23, 39, 65, 106, 121, 124, 129
neonatal, 109
nerve, 72
neuropathological, 72
neuropathologies, 1
neutral lipids, 68
neutrophil, 130
New York, 101
New Zealand, 10, 19, 104, 107
Nielsen, 120, 124
nitrate, 44
nitric oxide, 44, 47, 53, 57
nitrogen, 49, 50
nitrosative stress, 105
NMR, 128
nodulation, 76, 79
Norfolk, 111, 113, 115, 118, 121, 129
normal, 22, 63, 67, 69, 84
Norway, 10, 112
N-terminal, 58

nucleation, 62
nucleic acid, 40, 46, 48
nucleoprotein, 36
nucleotide sequencing, 31
nucleotides, 30, 35, 49, 85
nutrient (s), 22, 40, 43, 52, 68, 72, 88, 89, 91, 105, 108, 120

O

observations, 40, 41, 52, 89
obsolete, 7
offal, 24
oil (s), 15, 105
oligosaccharide, 72
online, 96, 108, 112, 118, 125, 133
operator, 64
operon, 29, 31, 64, 78, 80, 102, 132
oral, 20, 101
organelles, 68
organic, 14, 20, 21, 56, 87, 102, 110
organism, 23, 24, 42, 43, 48, 61, 64, 85
organization, 79, 122
organophosphates, 45
orientation, 36
osmotic, 39, 41, 42, 72, 93, 117
overproduction, 53
oviduct, 20
oxidation, 41, 43, 47, 49, 56, 58, 59, 96, 98, 105, 114
oxidative, 32, 41, 42, 44, 46, 48, 49, 50, 51, 52, 53, 54, 56, 57, 58, 60, 61, 62, 75, 90, 93, 97, 98, 99, 102, 103, 105, 109, 110, 113, 116, 118, 124, 126, 130, 131, 132
oxidative damage, 46, 52, 62, 103
oxidative stress, 32, 41, 46, 50, 51, 52, 53, 54, 56, 57, 58, 60, 61, 75, 93, 97, 98, 99, 102, 105, 109, 110, 116, 124, 126, 130, 131, 132
oxide (s), 47, 53, 57

oxygen, vii, 1, 5, 22, 32, 41, 44, 46, 47, 49, 50, 51, 52, 57, 58, 59, 60, 61, 91, 99, 106, 107, 111, 113, 118, 121, 123
Ozone, 47, 49

P

pain, 1
Pakistan, 113
paramagnetic, 106
Paris, 105, 121, 126
Parkinson, 107
pasteurization, 15
pathogenesis, 30, 32, 119
pathogenic, 16, 31, 46, 72, 83, 104, 110, 122
pathogens, vii, 30, 46, 62, 65, 78, 80, 97, 104, 110, 121, 132
pathways, vii, 1, 32, 49, 60, 75, 121
patients, 3, 23
pellicle, 89, 90
peptide, 105
peripheral nerve, 72
periplasm, 56, 68, 108
permeability, 77, 79, 120, 130
permit, 59, 64
peroxidation, 47, 48
peroxide, 46, 51, 52, 53, 56, 58, 59, 60, 100, 101, 106, 108, 121, 124, 133
personal communication, 24
perturbation, 49
pets, 9, 10, 20, 24
pH values, 14
phage, 8, 23, 30, 109, 113
phagocytic, 33
phenol, 109
phenotype (s), 43, 44, 78, 83, 85, 105, 107
phenotypic, 23, 43, 96, 113
phenylalanine, 116
phosphate, 13, 14, 16, 33, 44, 68, 77, 83, 86, 89, 90, 126, 127, 132
phosphatidylcholine, 68
phosphatidylserine, 68

phospholipids, 48, 49, 68, 74, 76
phosphonates, 45
phylogenetic, 30
phylogeny, 30
phylum, 4
physiological, 17, 22, 40, 41, 42, 43, 45, 63, 75, 86, 111
physiology, 16, 22, 45, 63, 67, 82, 109, 121
pig (s), 17, 18, 19, 96, 109, 122
plants, 34, 97
plasma membrane, 68
plasmid (s), 31, 34, 35, 36, 96, 97, 98, 111, 116, 120, 129, 132
plasticity, 23, 32, 33, 129
play, 42, 56, 57, 60, 63, 67, 72, 79, 82
point mutation, 23, 80, 100
poisoning, 1
policy makers, 20
pollutants, 72
polymer matrix, 87
polymerase, 23, 63, 128
polymerase chain reaction (PCR), 8, 18, 23, 31, 33, 84, 103, 128
polymorphism, 8, 23
polyphosphates, 44
polysaccharide, 29, 33, 34, 41, 62, 69, 72, 77, 89, 97
polystyrene, 89
polyunsaturated fatty acids, 48, 49
poor, 5, 23
population, 1, 3, 9, 12, 14, 23, 40, 50, 51, 106, 107
pore (s), 78, 101, 103
pork, 10, 24
portability, 9
post-translational, 45
potassium, 33
poultry, 9, 12, 16, 20, 23, 24, 25, 61, 72, 102, 104, 109, 110, 114, 115, 122, 131
power, 23
pregnant, 17
preparation, 11, 24
pressure, 11, 14, 30, 42, 58, 72, 75, 126, 133

prevention, 11, 120
prisoners, 3
probe, 124
product design, 108
production, 7, 12, 16, 25, 49, 53, 57, 83, 113, 119, 131
prokaryotes, 42, 72, 130
prokaryotic, 68
proliferation, 11, 12, 88
promote, 85, 113
promoter, 80, 131
property, 16
proteases, 63
protection, 2, 57, 77, 109, 116, 124, 131
protective role, 14
proteic, 16
protein (s), 7, 8, 29, 30, 33, 34, 35, 36, 41, 42, 43, 44, 46, 47, 48, 50, 52, 53, 54, 55, 56, 57, 58, 59, 60, 61, 63, 64, 68, 69, 70, 76, 78, 79, 80, 82, 83, 84, 85, 86, 87, 89, 90, 95, 96, 98, 99, 101, 103, 104, 106, 108, 111, 118, 120, 124, 132, 133
protein function, 47
protein oxidation, 48
protein sequence, 84
protein structure, 52, 106
protein synthesis, 43, 61, 101
proteins, 7, 29, 30, 33, 34, 35, 36, 41, 44, 46, 47, 48, 52, 53, 54, 56, 57, 58, 59, 60, 61, 63, 68, 76, 78, 83, 84, 85, 86, 87, 90, 95, 96, 108, 120, 131, 132, 133
proteobacteria, 4, 27, 64, 71, 98
proteome, 64, 96
protocol (s), 9, 12
protozoa, 22, 126
Pseudomonas, 84, 96, 109, 121
Pseudomonas aeruginosa, 96
public health, 93, 94
pulse, 23
pumps, 81, 107, 116
purification, 13, 128
pyrimidine, 49
pyruvate, 5, 86

Q

quinone (s), 118, 119, 122

R

radiation, 13, 100, 114
radical, 54, 55, 106
rainwater, 10
Random Amplified Polymorphism DNA (RAPD), 8
range, 1, 17, 20, 23, 24, 60, 63, 69, 73, 82, 91
raw materials, 11
reactive oxygen, 46, 47, 49, 59, 107, 118, 121
reactive oxygen species (ROS), 46, 47, 48, 50, 56, 57, 59, 107, 118
reactivity, 111
reading, 36
receptors, 86, 87
recognition, 85
recombination, 108
recontamination, 12
recovery, 22, 41, 129
recycling, 56, 60
red meat, 10, 13, 24
redox, 49, 51, 60, 124
reductases, 56, 60
reduction, 7, 11, 12, 14, 16, 20, 24, 42, 51, 52, 57, 70, 83
refrigeration, 12, 16
regular, 6
regulation (s), vii, 1, 12, 50, 52, 53, 54, 57, 60, 61, 64, 81, 82, 84, 91, 93, 97, 99, 103, 119, 121, 124, 130
regulators, 45, 58, 60, 80, 83, 93
relationship (s), 30, 109
relevance, 119, 121
repair, 30, 55, 57
reparation, 57
replacement, 131
replication, 29, 30, 35, 37, 132
repression, 44, 63

repressor, 58, 64, 80, 100
research, 59, 75, 83
researchers, 41
reserves, 44
reservoir (s), 9, 11, 16
residues, 35, 47, 59, 96
resistance, vii, 1, 12, 16, 25, 42, 43, 44, 46, 50, 51, 53, 56, 57, 58, 60, 62, 65, 68, 75, 76, 77, 78, 79, 80, 81, 82, 83, 93, 95, 97, 100, 101, 105, 107, 113, 115, 116, 117, 119, 120, 122, 123, 127, 129
resolution, 115, 128
respiration, 32, 44, 46, 130
respiratory, 32, 43, 45, 111
restaurant, 10
Restriction Fragment Length Polymorphism (RFLP), 8
resuscitation, 41, 102
retail, 24
reverse transcriptase, 128
Rhizobium, 34, 98
ribosomal, 29, 63, 90
ribosome, 35, 63
rings, 69
risk (s), 1, 10, 12, 16, 17, 19, 20, 22, 24, 25, 94, 111, 112, 120, 124
risk assessment, 124
risk factors, 10, 111, 120
risk management, 17
RNA, 29, 55, 60, 61, 63, 117, 124
RNAs, 37, 60, 110
rodent (s), 19, 20, 21
RRs, 82
rubber, 89
runoff, 24
Rutherford, 122

S

Saccharomyces cerevisiae, 30
safety, 5, 46, 115
salinity, 72
salmonella, 13, 62, 65, 78, 81, 84, 101, 103, 105, 107, 114, 118, 120, 127
salt (s), 40, 80, 115
sample, 13
saturated fatty acids, 70, 75
saturation, 73
scaffolding, 90
scanning electron microscopy, 105
scavenger, 118
Schmid, 126
search (es), 34, 63
seasonality, 18
secretion, 34, 35, 98
selectivity, 78, 79
self limiting, 25
sensing, 60, 94
sensitivity, 9, 13, 46, 49, 50, 58, 61, 65, 93, 94
sensor proteins, 83
sequencing, vii, 9, 27, 28, 29, 31, 61, 93
serine, 43, 68
serum, 69
severe stress, 52, 94
shape, 5
sheep, 17, 18, 19, 97, 117
shellfish, 10
shock, 41, 42, 43, 57, 58, 61, 62, 63, 64, 90, 93, 119, 126, 132
sialic acid, 72
signal transduction, 83, 86
signalling, 68, 121
similarity, 30, 31, 34, 35, 42, 93
sites, 35, 47, 69, 87, 106
Sjogren, 113
skin, 12, 24, 98
small intestine, 20, 21
small multidrug resistance (SMR), 76, 79, 81
sodium (NaCl), 5, 6, 16, 42, 83
soil (s), 17, 39
species, 4, 6, 7, 8, 11, 17, 18, 19, 21, 24, 27, 29, 40, 42, 43, 44, 46, 47, 49, 56, 59, 62, 71, 74, 88, 89, 95, 98, 102, 103, 106, 107, 109, 111, 116, 118, 119, 121, 124, 131

specificity, 32, 71, 101
spectra, 121
spectroscopy, 128
speed, 12, 18
spleen, 17
sporadic, 8, 9, 95, 106, 112, 120, 131
stability, 63, 106, 128
stabilization, 87
stages, 5
stainless steel, 89, 131
standardization, 9
Staphylococcus, 16, 105
Staphylococcus aureus, 16, 105
starvation, 39, 40, 41, 42, 43, 44, 45, 52, 58, 59, 62, 74, 93, 120, 129
steady state, 63
steel, 89, 131
sterile, 88
sterols, 68
stimulus, 82
stomach, 65
storage, 12, 45, 58, 59, 98, 131
strain (s), vii, 7, 8, 12, 13, 15, 16, 18, 19, 21, 22, 23, 24, 27, 30, 31, 32, 33, 34, 35, 40, 41, 43, 51, 56, 57, 61, 63, 64, 71, 72, 78, 80, 81, 84, 85, 89, 90, 95, 96, 98, 102, 103, 104, 110, 114, 119, 120, 122, 128
strategic, 20
strategies, 21, 24, 45, 46, 94, 95, 131
strength, 46
stress, vii, 1, 18, 32, 39, 42, 43, 44, 45, 46, 50, 51, 52, 53, 54, 56, 57, 58, 59, 60, 61, 62, 63, 64, 65, 72, 74, 75, 93, 95, 97, 98, 99, 102, 103, 105, 107, 109, 110, 111, 113, 116, 119, 120, 121, 124, 125, 126, 127, 128, 129, 130, 131, 132
substances, 15, 88, 91
substitution, 74
substrates, 48, 76, 79, 117
sugar, 7, 33, 49, 72
sulfate, 5
sulfur, 47, 48, 49
sulphur, 57

summer, 19, 21, 111
superoxide, 46, 47, 48, 50, 51, 52, 53, 54, 55, 58, 59, 62, 101, 106, 113, 119, 122, 126, 129
superoxide dismutase (SOD), 50, 52, 53, 55, 59, 60, 62, 101, 119, 122
supplements, 119
supply, 11, 88, 114, 118
suppression, 118
surface component, 69
surface properties, 30
surface structure, 63
surface water, 121
surveillance, 107
survivability, 22
survival, 12, 14, 15, 16, 17, 22, 23, 30, 39, 40, 41, 43, 44, 45, 51, 52, 53, 56, 58, 61, 62, 65, 67, 75, 88, 90, 91, 93, 98, 100, 103, 104, 105, 107, 112, 113, 117, 118, 119, 121, 123, 124, 126
susceptibility, 21, 53, 78, 79, 81, 97, 110, 114, 121
Sweden, 10, 113
Switzerland, 10, 126
symbiotic, 98
symptoms, 1
syndrome, 72, 125, 126
synthesis, 5, 31, 44, 61, 63, 68, 69, 71, 74, 89, 90, 99, 101, 106, 107, 124, 131
systematic review, 95
systems, vii, 7, 8, 21, 30, 41, 45, 47, 49, 50, 53, 54, 57, 60, 78, 79, 80, 81, 82, 84, 86, 88, 90, 94, 105, 115, 120, 131

T

targets, 49, 77
taxis, 86, 109
taxonomic, 6
taxonomy, 4
TCR, 45
tea, 15, 16, 103

temperature, 14, 19, 22, 34, 40, 41, 43, 61, 63, 72, 73, 74, 78, 79, 89, 93, 98, 99, 104, 119, 121
tension, 50, 52, 121
ternary complex, 87
tetracycline (s), 77, 80, 81, 129
thawing, 62
therapy, 115
thermal, 61, 63, 93, 113, 124
thermodynamic stability, 106
Thermophilic, 17, 120
thioredoxin, 55, 56, 57, 59, 60
Thomson, 108
threats, 91
time, 4, 7, 8, 13, 16, 19, 20, 40, 62, 63, 65, 88
tolerance, 46, 63, 65, 99, 102, 119
toxic, 5, 49, 69, 76, 79
toxicity, 52, 101, 106, 109, 113, 126
tracking, 25
traffic, 20
trans, 70, 73, 108, 109
transcriptase, 128
transcription, 29, 57, 59, 84, 114, 123
transcriptional, 64, 80, 81, 84, 96, 127, 133
transcripts, 64
transducer, 60, 86, 107, 133
transduction, 67, 83, 85, 86, 133
transfer, 36, 51
transformation, 12, 23, 52
transition, 46, 73, 74, 91
transition metal, 46
transition temperature, 73
translational, 90, 125
transmembrane, 67
transmission, 9, 19, 20, 22, 23, 30, 46, 72, 85, 96, 103, 110, 120
transparent, 6
transport, 11, 12, 18, 33, 34, 40, 41, 44, 47, 59, 63, 68, 90, 113, 127
transportation, 20, 90
transposons, 29, 34
travel, 10
trend, 61

tricarboxylic acid cycle, 44
tuberculosis, 123, 131
turgor, 42
turkeys, 19
tyrosine, 47

U

ubiquitous, 17, 21, 23
ultraviolet (UV), 13, 22, 40, 57, 100
unfolded, 63
United Kingdom, 10, 110, 113, 118, 121, 123, 133
United States, 3, 10, 14, 98, 106, 118
urban, 95
urease, 121
UV light, 57
UV radiation, 100

V

vaccination, 21, 103
vaccines, 20
vacuole, 33
vacuum, 15, 50, 104
Valencia, 129
values, 13, 14, 15, 62
vancomycin, 77
variability, 23, 31, 34, 78
variable, 12, 23, 30, 31, 33, 43, 78, 110, 112, 128
variation, 19, 23, 30, 63, 72, 78, 85, 127
vector, 9, 25, 96
veterinarians, 9
viable but nonculturable (VBNC), 5, 40, 41, 52, 60, 88, 93, 111
Vibrio cholerae, 74, 79, 84, 108, 123
virulence, vii, 1, 32, 37, 46, 63, 69, 72, 83, 97, 106, 107, 114, 117, 126, 133
viscosity, 126
visible, 6
visualization, 124

W

Wales, 24, 118
Washington, 10, 101, 106, 119, 121
waste, 24, 88
water, 10, 11, 12, 13, 14, 17, 20, 22, 24, 39, 41, 42, 45, 67, 72, 88, 100, 102, 104, 105, 114, 118, 129
Watson, 110
wild type, 64, 83
wildlife, 20
withdrawal, 9
workers, 9

Y

yield, 5, 34

Z

Zinc, 55
zoonotic, 22, 100